STUDY GUIDE TO ACCOMPANY

WHALEY & WONG'S

ESSENTIALS OF
Pediatric Nursing

FOURTH EDITION

Donna L. Wong
R.N., Ph.D., P.N.P., C.P.N., F.A.A.N.

By

Angela Ciolfi Murphy
R.N., M.S.N., Ph.D.

 **Mosby**

St. Louis Baltimore Boston Chicago London Madrid Philadelphia Sydney Toronto

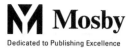
Mosby
Dedicated to Publishing Excellence

Executive Editor: Linda L. Duncan
Developmental Editor: Teri Merchant

*I wish to extend my appreciation to Donna Wong for her cooperation.
A special word of thanks to Regina Cabral for her editorial assistance
and to William, Brendan, Maia, and my parents for their support and
understanding during the writing of this study guide.*

SECOND EDITION

Printed in the United States of America

Mosby-Year Book, Inc.
11830 Westline Industrial Drive,
St. Louis, Missouri 63146

International Standard Book Number 0-8016-7415-8

95 96 97 GWM/P 9 8 7 6 5 4 3

Preface

Purpose

Whaley and Wong's Essentials of Pediatric Nursing by Donna L. Wong is a comprehensive textbook of pediatric nursing. This study guide is designed to facilitate the effective use of the textbook by students. Whereas the purpose of most study guides is to review chapter content, this manual has been designed not only to review content but also to enhance student learning through application exercises. The format affords the student the opportunity to apply the concepts of pediatric nursing to both traditional and nontraditional clinical settings employing the framework of the nursing process.

Organization

Each chapter in this manual is organized to incorporate all of the learning activities that will help students meet the objectives of the corresponding textbook chapter. The content of each chapter adheres to the following organizational pattern:

- *Chapter Overview* provides a brief synopsis of the major concepts and the focus of each textbook chapter.
- *Learning Objectives* define the expected learner outcomes and repeat those listed in the corresponding chapter of the textbook.
- *Review of Essential Concepts* provides students with an opportunity to assess their level of basic knowledge and comprehension.
- *Application, Analysis, and Synthesis of Essential Concepts* allow students the opportunity to apply knowledge of the chapter content to specific situations and clinical settings.
- *Suggested Readings* enable students to pursue appropriate resources for additional information.

The section entitled *Chapter Overview* highlights the major points addressed in each textbook chapter. The relevance of the content for students and the description of anticipated student learning outcomes are identified for each chapter.

The *Learning Objectives* section defines the expected knowledge that the student should have at the completion of the corresponding chapter.

The section entitled *Review of Essential Concepts* provides students with an opportunity to assess their knowledge and comprehension of the basic sciences and humanities, as well as chapter content. This is accomplished through the use of fill-in-the-blank, true/false, matching, and short answer questions.

The section entitled *Application, Analysis, and Synthesis of Essential Concepts* assists students in evaluating their knowledge of anatomy and physiology, developmental theories, and basic pathophysiology. This section bridges the gap between classroom theory and clinical application. It offers students an opportunity to apply the concepts obtained within the chapters to specific practicum settings. The nursing process serves as the organizational structure of this section. A learning technique called "Experiential Exercises" provides the student with an opportunity to gain structured information through a guided learning experience. The students should be able to answer the questions that follow the exercise; however, some of these settings are not universally available. If this difficulty arises, students should be able to complete the questions by using the book *Whaley and Wong's Essentials of*

Pediatric Nursing. Another learning technique used in this section is the "Clinical Situation." The student will be expected to answer questions related to actual care of the child and/or family. The questions related to these situations have a nursing focus. Students will be expected to assess the patient's health status, develop appropriate nursing diagnoses, identify pertinent nursing goals and interventions, and evaluate the effectiveness of the patient's plan of care.

The *Suggested Readings* section is composed of annotated readings that will serve as a resource to enhance knowledge gained from the textbook.

Conclusion

It is my hope that this manual, in conjunction with the fourth edition of *Whaley and Wong's Essentials of Pediatric Nursing*, will foster an innovative and effective approach to student learning.

Angela C. Murphy

Contents

Chapter 1
Perspectives of Pediatric Nursing

I. Chapter Overview

The content of Chapter I provides an overview of the nursing of children from a child-centered perspective that views children as unique individuals rather than miniature adults. The focus of care is on prevention of illness and promotion of health. At the completion of this chapter, the student should have a knowledge of the emerging trends in health care of children and their families. This knowledge will provide the basis from which students may approach contemporary health care issues of pediatric nursing.

II. Learning Objectives

Upon completion of this chapter, it is expected that the student will be able to:

1. Define the terms mortality and morbidity.

2. Identify two ways that knowledge of mortality and morbidity can improve child health.

3. List three major causes of illness during childhood.

4. Outline four events that were significant in the evolution of child health care in the United States.

5. Describe five broad functions of the pediatric nurse in promoting the health of children.

III. Review of Essential Concepts

1. The United States lags behind other countries of the world in infant mortality rate. In 1989, the United States ranked _____.

2. The country with the lowest infant mortality rate is _____.

3. The cause that accounts for 50% of the deaths of children less than 1 year of age in the United States is:
   a. cancer
   b. respiratory illness
   c. tonsillitis
   d. enuresis

4. The major cause of death for children over the age of 1 year is_____.

5. The_____ of the child partially determines the types of injuries that are most likely to occur.

6. The most significant event in the reduction of mortality in children in the United States was:
   a. the discovery and use of immunizations and antibiotics
   b. the development of the Maternal and Child Health Program
   c. the establishment of child labor laws
   d. the discoveries of Spitz and Robertson

7. The term *morbidity* is defined as:
   a. the number of individuals who have died over a specific period of time
   b. the prevalence of a specific illness in the population at a particular time

c. disease occurring with greater frequency than the number of expected cases in a community

d. disease occurring regularly within a geographic location

8. The most common childhood illness is:
   a. cancer
   b. respiratory illness
   c. tonsillitis
   d. enuresis

9. Behavioral, social, and educational problems are sometimes referred to as the _____.

10. The barriers to health care for children are _____ _____, _____ _____, _____ _____.

11. Nursing that involves 24-hours responsibility and accountability by one nurse for the care of a small group of patients is known as _____.

12. Identify the major roles of the pediatric nurse.
    a.

    b.

    c.

    d.

    e.

    f.

    g.

    h.

13. To effectively fulfill all aspects of the therapeutic role, the nurse must establish a _____ _____.

IV. Application, Analysis, and Synthesis of Essential Concepts

A. Experiential Exercise: Spend a morning at the Department of Health to survey the vital statistics affecting children in a given community.
   1. Define the following terms:
      a. Mortality--

      b. Morbidity--

2. How could the nurse utilize the mortality and morbidity statistics in a given community to improve child health?

3. What is the most effective approach to reducing morbidity and mortality?

B. Experiential Exercise: Spend a day following a nurse in a pediatric unit.
   1. Briefly describe and give examples of the eight broad functions of the pediatric nurse in a pediatric unit.
      a. Family Advocacy--

      b. Illness Prevention/Health Promotion--

      c. Health Teaching--

      d. Support/Counseling--

      e. Therapeutic Role--

      f. Coordination/Collaboration--

      g. Research--

      h. Health Care Planning--

   2. Describe the way in which primary nursing encourages professional accountability.

V. Suggested Readings

Folwer MD: Ethical decision making in clinical practice, Nurs Clin N Am 24(4):955, 1989.

> This article covers myriad facets of ethics. Beginning with a definition, the author then presents three subject matters of ethics. Approaches to ethical decision making (casuistic model and analytical model) are discussed in detail with illustrative examples. Dilemmas with suggestions for resolution are given. A useful and well-written article.

Laffrey S: Health promotion: relevance for nursing, Topics Clin Nurs 7(2):291-294, 1987.

> The author reviewed the research on definitions of health, health-related behaviors, and health promotion. The focus of the research was to learn more about the health potential of clients and how to promote that potential. Within nursing's broader definition of health, the nurse must be able to focus on the patient's definition of health and to learn to promote the health potential of the client. The author formulates a perspective from which nurses can assist the client to achieve the optimal level of health.

Nakamura RA and others: Excess infant mortality in an American Indian Population, 1940 to 1990, JAMA 2661(16):2244-2248, 1991.

> Infant mortality rates and causes for a typical native American community were analyzed. The Native American tribe of Warm Springs Indian Reservation in Oregon were the subjects. Causes of infant mortality and rates for the last 50 years were compared with the national average. Results showed that this tribe's rate of infant mortality was 2.6 times the national average and that sudden infant death syndrome accounted for almost all of the excess mortality since 1980. Implications for intervention and education are suggested.

Rushton CH: Ethical decision making in critical care, Part 1: The role of the pediatric nurse, Pediatr Nurs 14(5):411-412, 1988.

> For nurses working in neonatal or pediatric critical care settings, ethical questions assume significant proportions. The nurse in these settings is presented with dilemmas and conflicting loyalties. The role of pediatric nurses in ethical decision making is often ambiguous. Strategies for resolving ethical dilemmas are presented.

Chapter 2
Nursing Process in Care of the Child and Family

I. Chapter Overview

Chapter 2 defines and explains the nursing process, which is the framework for the practice of nursing. The process of assessment and the formulation and classification of the nursing diagnosis are discussed. The use of the nursing process in formulating standard and individualized nursing care plans is illustrated. At the completion of this chapter, the student will be able to utilize the nursing process to identify nursing diagnoses and formulate nursing care plans for both the child and his family.

II. Learning Objectives

Upon completion of this chapter, it is expected that the student will be able to:

1.   List the five steps of the nursing process.

2.   Differentiate among different types of assessment: comprehensive, screening, and focused.

3.   Differentiate among three domains of nursing practice: dependent, independent, and interdependent.

4.   Define nursing diagnosis.

5.   Describe the five steps in developing a goal/outcome.

6.   Differentiate standard nursing care plan from individualized plan of care.

III. Review of Essential Concepts

1. List the five steps of the nursing process.
    a.

    b.

    c.

    d.

    e.

2. Define the following three levels of assessment:
    a. Comprehensive–

    b. Screening–

    c. Focused–

3. Gordon's _____ categories of _____ _____ may be utilized as the framework to assess the child and his family.

4. List the eleven functional health patterns in Gordon's framework:
    a.

    b.

    c.

d.

e.

f.

g.

h.

i.

j.

k.

5. Differentiate among three domains of nursing practice: dependent, independent, and interdependent.
   a.

   b.

   c.

6. Nursing diagnosis should reflect the _____ and _____ dimensions of nursing practice.
7. The three components of nursing diagnosis are:
   a.

   b.

   c.

8. Match each of the following definitions with the appropriate term.
   a. ___ problem
   b. ___ etiology
   c. ___ signs and symptoms
      1) the child's response to health pattern deficits in the child, family, or community
      2) cluster of cues and/or defining characteristics that are derived from patient assessment
      3) physiologic, situational, and maturational factors that cause the problem or influence its development
9. In the planning stage of the nursing process _____ or _____ are established.

10. Describe the five steps in developing a goal/outcome.
    a.

    b.

    c.

    d.

    e.

11. Define the two types of nursing care plans.
    a. Standard care plans—

    b. Individualized care plans—

12. The implementation phase of the nursing process is defined as:

13. Comparison of the expected outcomes against observed behavior is the final stage of the nursing process; this stage is termed _____.

IV. Application, Analysis, and Synthesis of Essential Concepts

A. Experiential Exercise: Spend a day following a nurse in a pediatric unit.
   1. In order to complete a comprehensive assessment of one of the children and her parent, the nurse will systematically collect data from what possible sources?
      a.

      b.

      c.

      d.

      e.

      f.

2. The nurse identifies that the child is experiencing difficulty lying comfortably in a supine position because of pain from an abdominal incision.
   a. The appropriate nursing diagnosis to identify this problem would be located in which functional category?

   b. State the nursing diagnosis that describes this child's response.

   c. What is the "problem" in this diagnostic statement?

   d. What is the "etiology" in this nursing diagnosis?

   e. What are the signs and symptoms for this nursing diagnosis?

3. State an appropriate goal for the above nursing diagnosis.

4. State one intervention for the above goal.

5. State one criterion for evaluation of the above goal.

B. Experiential Exercise: Spend a morning in a pediatric unit and complete a comprehensive assessment of one child and his family.
   1. Identify whether the following characteristic of "assessment" describes a standardized or individualized care plan.
      Information is specific to both identified problem and the child and family.

   2. Identify whether the following characteristic of "nursing diagnosis" describes a standardized or individualized care plan.
      All probable nursing diagnoses with general etiologic factors are considered.

   3. Identify whether the following characteristic of "planning" describes a standardized or individualized care plan.

Goals are specific and reflect patient outcomes.

4. Identify whether the following characteristic of "implementation" describes a standardized or individualized care plan.
   Nursing interventions are specific and provide direction for nursing care of individual patient.

5. Identify whether the following characteristic of "evaluation" describes a standardized or individualized care plan.
   Progress the patient is expected to make is identified.

V. Suggested Reading

Gordon M: Nursing diagnoses and the diagnostic process, Am Nurs 76(8):1298-1300, 1976.

In this classic article Marjory Gordon describes the concept of nursing diagnosis and the diagnostic process. Diagnostic categories, their components, and the diagnostic statement is explained according to Gordon's thesis. Though the process has been refined in the intervening years, the foundation set in this article remains firm.

Rhodes AM: Contents of nurses' detailed notes, MCN 12(3):61, 1987.

The record on nursing observations and nursing care is a critical part of every patient's medical history. The author describes what information should be documented by nurses regarding: assessment, nursing intervention, health teaching, accountability information, and diagnostic tests. The goal of charting should be to provide the most concise yet complete information on patients to ensure continuity of care and to protect against any legal questions.

Shamansky S, Yanni CR: In opposition to nursing diagnoses: a minority opinion, Image 15(2):47-50, 1983.

This article examines the premises underlying nursing diagnoses and their impact on clinicians and the health care delivery system. The authors argue that nursing diagnoses in their current form limit nursing practice, create obstacles to clear communication, and constrain inference and intuition.

Chapter 3

Social, Cultural, and Religious Influences on Child Health Promotion

I. Chapter Overview

Chapter 3 provides an overview of the cultural, social, religious, and economic factors influencing the growth and development of children in the United States. The influence of religious and cultural beliefs on health care practices is discussed at length. The effect of the nurse's own cultural beliefs on the delivery of nursing care is explored. At the completion of this chapter, the student will have a knowledge of the social, economic, cultural and religious influences that affect the health promotion of the child. This orientation will enable the student to adapt the delivery of nursing care to the unique needs of the child and his family.

II. Learning Objectives

Upon completion of this chapter, it is expected that the student will be able to:

1. Define culture, culture shock, ethnicity, and race.

2. Describe the subcultural influences on child development in the areas of socialization, education, and aspiration.

3. Compare and contrast the advantages and disadvantages encountered in the educational system by children from lower- and middle-class backgrounds.

4. Characterize family life in present-day America.

5. Identify four common diseases or disorders that affect certain ethnic or cultural groups.

6. Identify areas of potential conflict of values and customs for a nurse interacting with a family from a different cultural/ethnic group.

7. Describe three religious groups whose beliefs significantly affect their health practices.

III. Review of Essential Concepts

1. Match each of the following concepts with the appropriate definition.
    a. ___ culture
    b. ___ race
    c. ___ ethnicity
    d. ___ socialization
    1) the process by which children acquire the beliefs, values, and behaviors of a given society
    2) the way of life a group of people develop to adapt to their physical or social circumstances
    3) the affiliation of a set of persons who share a unique cultural, social, and linguistic heritage
    4) a division of mankind possessing traits that are transmissible by descent and sufficient to characterize it as a distinct human type
2. A social group consists of a system or roles carried out in both primary and secondary groups.

a. A primary group is characterized by:

b. A secondary group is characterized by:

3. The subcultures that seem to exert the greatest influence on childrearing are _____, _____, _____, and_____.
4. Define ethnicity.

5. The greatest influence on childrearing practices and their consequences is the _____ of the family into which a child is born.
6. Identify the major educational disadvantages encountered by lower-class children.
   a.

   b.

   c.

   d.

   e.

   f.

7. The term "visible poverty" refers to:

8. The term "invisible poverty" refers to:

9. Homelessness is particularly damaging for _____ age children.
10. _____ families are subject to inadequate sanitation, substandard housing, social isolation, and lack of educational and medical facilities.
11. Identify four functions of the peer subculture.
    a.

    b.

c.

d.

12. Family life in America is characterized by a pervasive sense of _____, increasing _____ and _____ mobility. Children in America grow up with a number of adults who provide _____ to them as _____ models. Most children live in some form of _____ family in sharply differentiated _____.
13. Define "cultural shock."

14. Match the following common diseases or disorders with the ethnic or cultural group they affect:
    a. ___ tuberculosis
    b. ___ Tay-Sachs disease
    c. ___ cystic fibrosis
    d. ___ sickle cell disease
       1) Ashkenasi Jewish
       2) Blacks
       3) Whites
       4) Native Americans of Southwest, Vietnamese, Mexican-Americans
15. The nurse should know about the _____, _____, and _____ of other ethnic groups in order to meet the needs of the families and to gain their cooperation and compliance in health care.
16. _____ is the concept that any behavior must be judged first in relation to the context of the culture in which it occurs.
17. Identify the areas in which there might be a conflict of values and customs for the nurse interacting with a child and family from a different cultural or ethnic group.
    a.

    b.

    c.

    d.

    e.

    f.

    g.

h.

i.

j.

k.

l.

m.

n.

18. Identify three religious groups whose beliefs significantly affect their health practices.
    a.

    b.

    c.

IV. Application, Analysis, and Synthesis of Essential Concepts

A. Experiential Exercise: Interview parents from a variety of cultural, ethnic, economic, and religious backgrounds to determine the differences in childrearing practices. Answer the following questions and include specific parental responses that illustrate the concepts.
   1. Briefly describe the impact the cultural and subcultural factors have on growth and development.

   2. What are some of the subcultural influences that may affect this family's childrearing practices?
      a.

      b.

      c.

      d.

      e.

      f.

      g.

3. Briefly describe the influence that the following aspects of contemporary American culture have on child development.
   a. An optimistic view of the world and belief that things can be better—

   b. Increasing geographic and economic mobility—

   c. A basically nuclear-family orientation—

   d. Influence of multiple adults—

   e. Schools—

B. Experiential Exercise: Spend a day in a health care center that serves a multicultural community. Answer the following questions and include specific observations as appropriate.
   1. What factors increase a child's susceptibility to health problems?
      a.

      b.

   2. How do the following factors contribute to the development of health problems in children from lower socioeconomic classes?
      a. Inadequate funds for food—

      b. Lack of funds and access to health care—

c. Poor sanitation and crowded living conditions—

3. Why should nurses working in a multicultural community be aware of their own attitudes and values?

4. What two areas of religious belief should be evaluated when assessing health care practices?
a.

b.

5. Describe three ways in which the nurse can incorporate ethnic practices into effective health care delivery.
a.

b.

c.

C. Experiential Exercise: Spend a morning in each of two preschool programs: one that focuses on children from middle-class backgrounds and one that focuses on children from the lower socioeconomic backgrounds. Observe the children's interactions with the teachers and with each other and answer the following questions. Include examples of behavior that confirm your conclusions.
1. Orientation to time—

2. Parental expectations—

3. Communication skills—

V.   Suggested Readings

Anderson JM: Health care across cultures, Nurs Outlook 38(3):136-138, 1990.

> This author purports that sociocultural variations influence (1) the subjective experiences of health and illness of the client and (2) how clients seek and comply with help. If the nurse does not recognize these variations and adjust the care, then this omission will become an obstacle to care. The author offers a negotiation model by which nurses can determine patients' perceptions of their illness and adjust care so that it is culturally acceptable to the patients and their families.

Bassuk EL, Rosenberg L: Psychosocial characteristics of homeless children and children with homes, Pediatrics 85(3):257-261, 1990.

> This study made a comparison of 86 children from 49 homeless Boston families headed by women and 134 children from 81 housed Boston families headed by women. In both groups the mothers were poor, single, and receiving welfare payments. The data indicated that many homeless children and poor children have severe problems. A higher proportion of homeless children displayed developmental delay and depression. Both homeless and poor children had worse scores on anxiety measures than comparison groups. The ability to function will be severely hampered in these children unless prevention measures are undertaken.

Lawson L: Culturally sensitive support for grieving parents, MCN 15(2):76-79, 1990.

> The author focused on the following cultures: Native American, Mexican-Americans, and Southeast Asians. The cultural beliefs of each of these groups affect the grieving of these parents following the death of their infant. Specific cultural influences on how members of a family grieve are presented. A detailed cultural assessment is explained. Specific cultural beliefs regarding family life, religion and healing, death and grief, and interaction with health professionals are presented for each of the three cultural groups. The author concludes by citing nursing implications for culturally sensitive care. An annotated bibliography is listed for further study. An excellent reference for any student caring for these cultural groups.

Niederhauser VP: Health care of immigrant children: incorporating culture into practice, Pediatr Nurs 15(6):569-674, 1989.

As the title implies, this article delineates how the nurse can incorporate culture into the care of clients. Culture plays a major role in health care and especially in compliance. A comprehensive cultural assessment tool is included for the use of the nurse. It is emphasized that in order for nurses to deliver culturally sensitive care, they need to understand themselves and their own cultural values as well as those of the client.

Rosenburg JA: Health care for Cambodian children: integrating treatment plans, Pediatr Nurs 12:118-125, 1986.

This article explores the health beliefs and health practices of Cambodian families. The information in this article will help the nurse to assess the health beliefs of the Cambodian children and their families. Incorporating the health beliefs and practices into nursing care plans will enhance client compliance and improve relationships between health-care providers and these families.

Van Breda A: Health issues facing Native American children, Pediatr Nurs 15(6):575-577, 1989.

The current health status of Native American children is inseparable from the problems of the Native American society at large. The dominant issues for these children are poverty and alcoholism. Three major nursing implications for the nurse involved with this population are presented and explained.

Chapter 4

Family Influences On
Child Health Promotion

I.   Chapter Overview

The overall description and purpose of the family is explored in Chapter 4. Family theories and different family structures are explored. The role transition of new parents and the effect of family size on personality development are discussed. Parenting behaviors and special parenting situations are explored. Since families assume the primary responsibility for childrearing and socialization, students need to be aware of the impact of the family on the developing child. At the completion of this chapter, the student will have knowledge of a variety of parenting situations that will serve as a foundation for the development of appropriate nursing strategies.

II.   Learning Objectives

Upon completion of this chapter, it is expected that the student will be able to:

1.   Discuss definitions of family.

2.   Describe two major family theories.

3.   Identify different family structures found in the United States.

4.   Discuss the effect of family size and configuration on personality development.

5.   Discuss the role transition experienced by new parents.

6.   Explain various parenting behaviors such as

parenting styles, disciplinary patterns, and communication skills.

7.   Demonstrate an understanding of special parenting situations such as adoption, divorce, single parenting, step-parenting, and dual-career families.

III. Review of Essential Concepts

1.   State and explain the three major family theories.
     a. *Family System Theory - acts with members and environment (interaction)*

     b. *Developmental Theory - family Life cycle approach to compare families at various stages of development.*

     c. *Family Stress Theory - How families react to stressful events and suggest factors that promote adaptation*

2.   List the three major objectives of the family in relation to children:
     a. *caregiving*

     b. *nurturing*

     c. *training*

3. Match the following family structures with the appropriate definition.
   a. _4_ nuclear
   b. _2_ single parent
   c. _5_ reconstituted
   d. _1_ extended
   e. _3_ alternative family
   1) the nuclear family, plus lineal or collateral relatives
   2) a man or woman alone as head of household as a result of divorce, death, desertion, illegitimacy, or adoption
   3) polygamy, communal family, homosexual family
   4) a man, his wife, and their children who live in a common household
   5) married adults, one or both of whose children from a previous marriage reside in the household

4. Roles are learned through the _socialization_ process.

5. Identify the four elements of family configuration that influence child development.
   a. _family size_
   b. _spacing of children_
   c. _ordinal position in family_
   d. _sibling interaction_
   e. _multiple births_

6. To differentiate between small and large family configurations, decide if the following statements are true or false.
   a. _T_ Emphasis is placed on the individual development of the child in the small family.
   b. _F_ Children in large families are unable to adjust to a variety of changes and crises.
   c. _F_ Children's development and achievement is measured against other children in the neighborhood in the large family.
   d. _T_ Adolescents from a large family are often more peer oriented than family oriented.

7. Identify the three basic goals of parenting.
   a. _Physical survival and health of children._
   b. _Skills + abilities necessary to be a self-sustaining adult_
   c. _behavioral capabilities for maximizing cultural values and beliefs._

8. Briefly identify the five factors that can influence the parental role.
   a. _parental age + previous experience_
   b. _father involvement_
   c. _effects of stress_
   d. _characteristics of the infant_
   e. _marital relationship_

9. Differentiate among the following three styles of parental control.
   a. authoritarian— _strict rules + regulations_
   b. permissive— _lets child make decision viewing themselves as resources, not role model_

   (combination of the two)

   c. authoritative— _guides child behavior + attitude by emphasizing the need for rules negative reinforcement deviation_

10. Identify the five most common strategies for discipline.
   a. _spanking_
   b. _time out_
   c. _behavioral modification_
   d. _reasoning + scolding_
   e. _consequences_

11. Match the following guidelines for implementing discipline with their explanations.
   a. _3_ consistency
   b. _6_ timing
   c. _1_ commitment
   d. _5_ flexibility
   e. _2_ behavior orientation
   f. _4_ termination
   1) follow through with the details of discipline
   2) always disapprove of the behavior, not the child
   3) implement disciplinary action exactly as agreed upon for each infraction
   4) once the discipline is administered, consider the child has having a "clean slate"

5) choose disciplinary strategies that are appropriate to the child's temperament and the severity of the misbehavior

6) initiate discipline as soon as the child misbehaves

12. ___ Almost half the adoptable children in the United States are adopted by relatives. (true or false)

13. State the two areas of concern for adoptive parents.

a. Telling the child he's adopted.

b. Adolescents may use adoption as tool in defying authority.

14. Identify the factors that will influence the impact of divorce on children.

a. age + sex of children

b. outcome of divorce

c. quality of parental care following divorce

15. ___ It has been determined that at least half the children in the United States spend some time in a single-parent home (true or false).

16. List the five guidelines for step-parenting.

a. Let relationship develop slowly

b. Don't criticize or belittle loss parents or erase them

c. Expect confused feelings, anxiety competition for attention, bids for loyalty

d. Communicate

e. Get help if needed

IV. Application, Analysis, and Synthesis of Essential Concepts

A. Experiential Exercise: After talking with children from a variety of families, answer the following questions that deal with the effects of different family structures on child development. Include specific examples to illustrate these concepts.

1. Define family structure. Individuals w/ socially recognized statuses + positions who interact w/ one another on a regular basis.

2. What events might alter family structure? marriage, divorce, birth, death, abandonment, incarceration.

3. What implication does an alteration in composition have for the family and child? Roles must be redefined or redistributed.

4. What are the advantages and/or disadvantages of the following types of family structure?

a. Nuclear— Highly adaptable. Ability to adjust + reshape when needed. Free to move + not dependent on cooperation from other members. Where wide geographic separation, parents + no relatives for advice, assistance or child care.

b. Single-parent— liberal attitudes made possible to rear children w/ one parent. Frequently children in this family are reared into extended families.

c. Extended— More functional where land basis of wealth + substance. Basic social educational + productive unit. Needs of individual are sublimated for welfare of family.

B. Experiential Exercise: Talk to a single parent to assess problem areas. Answer the following questions and include specific parental responses.

1. What changes or feelings accompany single parenthood? Altered self-image; need for realignment of role, feel of anger, remorse, guilt, retaliation and sorrow for oneself.

2. Describe the impact of single parenting on the child. Parent devote more attention to child because of feeling guilt + low self esteem. Children feel the burden of parents happiness is on their shoulders.

3. Identify some of the major problems associated with dual-career families. Stress is both economic + emotional Fatigue + erratic parenting occur, lonliness

4. What factors influence the effect of a mother's absence from the home?

a. age of child

b. attitude of the father towards the wife absence

c. *regularity with which the mother is away from home*

d. *availability and quality of substitute child care.*

C. Experiential Exercise: Interview an expectant couple and parents with adolescent children to contrast their views of parenthood. Answer the following questions and include the parents' responses to illustrate these concepts.

1. What types of motivation may enter into a decision to initiate a pregnancy?

    a. *assomption that all normal people get married + have children*

    b. *proof of biologic adequacy + demonstration of adulthood.*

    c. *fulfills a parents wish for grand-children + perpetuate the family name + fortune*

    d. *attempt to save a tenous marriage.*

2. According to Duvall's Development Stages of the Family Theory, what are the tasks for each of these families? Are these families successful in accomplishing these tasks?

    a. Expectant couple— *Integrate infants into family. accomodate to new parenting + grandparenting. Maintain marital bond.*

    b. Parents of adolescent children—
    Adolescents develop autonomy. Parents refocus on midlife marital + career issues. Parents begin a shift for older generation

3. What factors influence the way in which parents rear their children?
    Cultural influences, social class, and economic resources.

V. Suggested Readings

Arditti JA: Noncustodial fathers: an overview of policy and resources, Family Relations 10:460-465, 1990.

Noncustodial fathers have been understudied in the social science literature. This article presents an overview of the literature and major policy issues relating to the following topics: child support, visitation, custody, and policy implications. Resources are identified that would be useful to professionals who are working with divorced fathers and their families.

Bray JH, Berger SH: Noncustodial father and paternal grandparent relationships in stepfamilies, Family Relations 10:414-419, 1990.

Ninety-eight children (ages 6-14) and their families were followed for seven years of a remarriage after divorce. Associations between the children's psychological adjustment in stepfather families and their relationship with their noncustodial fathers and paternal grandparents were studied. Differences in these relationships and how these relationships vary for boys and girls were investigated. Some controversial results are presented. Further longitudinal research is suggested.

Koepke JE, and others: Becoming parents: feelings of adoptive mothers, Pediatr Nurs 17(4):333-336, 1991.

To determine whether the feelings and reactions of adoptive mothers are any different from those of birth mothers, 24 adoptive mothers and 24 birth mothers were interviewed. The primary results indicated that the adoptive mothers were less prepared for motherhood then were the birth mothers. Nursing implications for education and counseling of the adoptive mothers are presented.

Melnyk BM: Changes in parent-child relationships following divorce, Pediatr Nurs 17(4):337-341, 1991.

Divorce imposes multiple stressors that disrupt parent-child relationships. The author explores the major factors influencing changes in the parent-child relationship, changes in mother-child relationships, changes in father-child relationships, and child outcomes following changes in parent-child relationships. Nursing intervention focuses on early intervention in the divorce process. Critical areas of assessment and intervention with both parents and children are discussed.

Wallace PM, Gotlib IH: Marital adjustment during the transition to parenthood: Stability and predictors of change, Marriage Fam 52:21-28, 1990.

Changes in marital adjustment following the birth of the first child were examined in a longitudinal study of 97 couples. A number of variables were identified as possible predictors of marital adjustment. Implications of the results of the study are discussed and suggestions for future research are offered.

Chapter 5

Developmental Influences on Child Health Promotion

I. Chapter Overview

Chapter 5 provides an overview of the physiologic, psychologic, environmental, and social factors influencing the growth and development process. In order to be able to promote optimal health and development of both child and family, students need to understand how children grow and interact with their environment. Upon completion of this chapter, students should be aware of the theoretical foundations of all areas of development. This knowledge will serve as a basis for nursing interventions to meet the complex needs of the developing child.

II. Learning Objectives

Upon completion of this chapter, it is expected that the student will be able to:

1. Describe major trends in growth and development.

2. Explain the alterations in the major body systems that take place during the processes of growth and development.

3. Discuss the development and relationships of cognitive, language, personality, moral, spiritual, and self-concept development.

4. Demonstrate an understanding of the role of innate and environmental factors in the physical and emotional development of children.

5. Describe the role of play in the growth and development of children.

III. Review of Essential Concepts

1. Match the following terms with their correct definitions:
    a. _3_ growth
    b. _1_ maturation
    c. _2_ development
    d. _4_ differentiation
    1) an increase in competence, adaptability, and aging
    2) a gradual growth and expansion involving a change from a lower to more advanced stage of complexity.
    3) an increase in number and size of cells as they divide and synthesize new proteins; results in increased size and weight of the whole or any of its parts
    4) a biologic description of the processes by which early cells and structure are modified and altered to achieve specific, characteristic physical and chemical properties

2. Fill in the ages denoted by each of the following periods of development.
    a. prenatal period– *conception – birth*

    b. neonatal period– *birth – 1month*

    c. infancy– *1month – 12months*

    d. early childhood– *1yr – 6yr*

e. toddler period– *1–3 yrs*

f. preschool period– *3yrs– 6yrs*

g. middle childhood or school age– *6yrs – 11 yrs*

h. adolescence– *12–18 yrs*

3. List the three directional trends in growth and development.
   a. *cephalocaudal, head-to-toe*
   b. *proximodistal, near-to-far*
   c. *mass to specific, differentiation*

4. Those times in the lifetime of an organism when it is more vulnerable to positive or negative influences are called *sensitive periods*.

5. For each of the following stages of development, match the body part in which growth predominates.
   a. *2* prenatal
   b. *1* infancy
   c. *4* early and middle
   d. *3* adolescence
      1) trunk
      2) head
      3) shoulder and hip breadth
      4) legs

6. The most prominent feature of childhood and adolescence is *physical growth*.

7. *F* Lymphoid tissue follows a growth pattern that is similar to that of other body tissues. (true or false)

8. The basal caloric requirement for infants is about *108* kcal/kg of body weight and decreases to *40* to *45* kcal/kg at maturity.

9. Identify the temperamental category that is described by each of the following.
   a. Highly active, irritable, and irregular in habits; adapts slowly to routines, people, situations–
   Difficult child

   b. Reacts negatively and with mild intensity to new stimuli; quite inactive and moody but shows only moderate irregularity in functions–
   slow-to warm up child

c. Even-tempered, regular, and predictable in habits; has positive approach to new stimuli; open and adaptable to change–
Easy child

10. List the five stages of psychosexual development and the ages encompassed by each.
    a. *oral –birth-yr*
    b. *anal – 1–3yrs*
    c. *phallic- 3-6yrs*
    d. *Latency – 6-12yrs*
    e. *genital –12yrs+over*

11. For each of the following age groups, identify Erikson's stage of psychosocial development.
    a. Birth to 1 year– *Trust vs. mistrust*

    b. 1 to 3 years– *autonomy vs shame and doubt*

    c. 3 to 6 years– *initiative vs. guilt*

    d. 6 to 12 years– *industry vs inferiority*

    e. 12 to 18 years– *identity vs. role confusion*

12. Match the following stages of cognitive development with the appropriate defining characteristics (answers may be used more than once; more than one answer may apply).
    a. *3,5* sensorimotor stage
    b. *1,8* preoperational stage
    c. *4,7* concrete operations
    d. *2,6* formal operations
       1) predominant characteristic is egocentricity
       2) thought is characterized by adaptability and flexibility
       3) progression from reflex activity to imitative behavior
       4) thought becomes increasingly logical and coherent; conservation is developed; problems are solved in a concrete, systematic fashion
       5) child begins to develop a sense of self as he differentiates self from environment

6) can think in abstract terms, use abstract symbols, and draw logical conclusions

7) child considers points of view other than his own; thinking becomes socialized

8) child is unable to see things from any perspective other than his own; thinking is concrete

13. Identify the stage of moral development that is described by each of the following statements.

a. Children conform to rules imposed by authority figures and are culturally oriented to the labels of good/bad and right/wrong.

Preconventional morality

b. Children endeavor to define moral values and principles that are agreed upon by the entire society. Emphasis is on the possibility for changing law in terms of societal needs.

postconventional level

c. Children are concerned with conformity and loyalty, actively maintaining, supporting, and justifying the social order.

Conventional level

14. Match the following types of play with their defining characteristics.
a. __2__ solitary play
b. ____ cooperative play   *Play is organized and children play in a group with other children*
c. __1__ onlooker play
d. ____ associative play   *Children play together but no organization*
e. __3__ parallel play

1) child watches what other children are doing but makes no attempt to enter into the play activity

2) child plays alone and independently with toys different from those of other children within the same area

3) child plays independently among other children with toys that are like those that the children around him are using, neither influencing nor being influenced by

15. __T__ Probably the single most important influence on growth is nutrition. (true or false)

16. The most prominent feature of emotional deprivation, particularly during the first year, is ___*developmental retardation*___.

17. List seven specific goals that play serves to develop throughout childhood.
a. *sensorimotor development*
b. *intellectual development*
c. *socialization*
d. *creativity*
e. *self-awareness*
f. *therapeutic value*
g. *moral value*

18. Children on long-term corticosteroid therapy will exhibit __*growth*__ __*retardation*__

19. Stress in childhood has been defined as:

an imbalance between environmental demands and a person's coping resources that disrupts the equilibrium of the person.

20. List six detrimental effects of protracted television viewing on children.
a. *increased verbally + physical aggressive behavior.*
b. *reduced persistence at problem solving.*
c. *greater sex role stereotyping*
d. *reduced creativity*
e. *linked to obesity and high blood cholesterol level*
f. *implicit messages that promote alcohol consumption, smoking, violence and promiscuous sexual activity.*

IV. **Application, Analysis, and Synthesis of Essential Concepts**

A. Experiential Exercise: Observe a child from each age group: infant, toddler, preschool, school-age, and adolescent.

1. Why is it necessary to have an understanding of patterns of development before assessing a child's developmental status?

Children vary in growth + development but certain predictable patterns are universal and basic to all human beings

2. Match the following developmental characteristics to the age groups in which they occur. (Answers may be used more than once; more than one answer may apply.)
   a. _4_ infant
   b. _1,2_ toddler
   c. _2,3_ preschooler
   d. _2_ school-age child
   e. _1,5_ adolescent
   1) 50% of adult height attained
   2) yearly weight gain of 2 to 3 kg
   3) birth length doubled
   4) rapid growth of trunk
   5) growth increase

3. Identify the psychosocial conflict of each age group and provide a specific intervention that will assist in the resolution of this conflict. (Erickson)
   a. infant– *Trust vs. Mistrust*
   Meet child needs
   provide loving care

   b. toddler– *autonomy vs. shame + doubt*
   Allow the child to make choices.

   c. preschool– *initiative vs. guilt*
   Encourage exploration of environment
   Set realistic limits.

   d. school-age– *industry vs. inferiority*
   Encourage competition + cooperation
   Assist in setting achievable goals

   e. adolescent– *Identity vs role confusion*
   Provide positive feedback regarding appearance and activity

4. What behavior might be observed in each age group that would indicate the level of spiritual development?
   a. infant– *no concept of right or wrong evident.*

   b. toddler– *imitation of religious gestures + behaviors of others without comprehensions of meaning.*

   c. preschool– *imitation of religious behavior and following of parental religious beliefs as part of daily lives without real understanding of concepts.*

   d. school-age– *strong interest in religion with acceptance of a diety, petitions to this diety made and expected to be answered.*

   e. adolescent– *realization that prayers are not always answered. Modification or abandonment of religious practices. Questioning of the religious standards of parents*

B. Experiential Exercise: Interview the parents of a newborn regarding the infant's temperament.
   1. What is the significance of assessing a child's temperament?
   Difficult to slow to warm patterns of behavior are more vulnerable to development of behavioral problems in early + middle childhood. Parents unable to accept + deal w/ childs behavior there is greater likelihood of subsequent behavioral problems.

   2. Identify behavioral characteristics that would indicate the temperament pattern of each of the following children.
   a. the easy child– *even tempered, regular + predictable habits, positive approach to new stimuli, adaptable to change*

   b. the difficult child– *highly active, irritable, irregular in habits, has negative withdrawal responses, slow to adapt to new routines, people or situations*

   c. the slow-to-warm-up child– *inactive, moody, moderately irregular in function, passively resistent to novelty or changes in routine, reacts neg with mild intensivety to new stimuli but reacts slowly w/ repeated contact*

C. Experiential Exercise: Attend a PTA meeting at your local elementary school. If you are asked to cite guidelines related to TV viewing for this age child, what guidelines would you present to this group?
   a. *Positive role model by developing television substitutes (reading, athletes, hobbies)*
   b. *Construct a time chart of childs activity*
   c. *Discuss what is balanced set of activities*
   d. *Select Appropriate TV shows at beginning of week.*
   e. *Allow child to select programs from approved list*
   f. *Limit childs viewing to 2 hrs or less per day.*
   g. *Rule out TV at specific times*
   h. *Make a list of alternate activities.*

V. Suggested Readings

Goldsmith M: Youngsters dialing up cholesterol levels, JAMA 264(23):2976, 1990.

> This author found a correlation between television viewing and high blood cholesterol levels in young persons 2 to 20 years of age. Excessive TV viewing was identified as a superior predictor in heart disease risk factor screening.

Gortmaker S, and others: Inactivity, diet, and the fattening of America, Am Dietetic Assoc 90(9):1247-1255, 1990.

> The study reported in this article identified television viewing as a strong risk factor for childhood and adolescent obesity, and documented an association between television viewing and obesity among adults. Inactivity, and increased intake were correlated factors. Multiple intervention approaches are necessary to prevent obesity.

Singer DG, editor: Children, adolescents, and television—1989. I. Television violence: critique, Pediatrics 83(3):445-446, 1989.

> The author reviewed the results of a number of studies that investigated the relationship of television viewing of violence and physical aggression. The studies confirmed that viewing violence on television increases aggressive behaviors in the child.

Chapter 6

Communication and Health Assessment of the Child and Family

I. Chapter Overview

Chapter 6 introduces an essential component of the nursing of children and their families, communication. It is important because it is an essential skill in the assessment process and may be crucial to the establishment of a trusting relationship with children and their families. Guidelines for taking a health history are presented. Family, home, and nutritional assessment is explored. At the completion of this chapter, the student should have knowledge of the communication process with children and their families and will be able to apply this knowledge to the care of children and their families in the clinical area.

II. Learning Objectives

Upon completion of this chapter, it is expected that the student will be able to:

1. Describe guidelines for communication and interviewing.

2. Identify communication strategies for interviewing parents.

3. Formulate guidelines for using an interpreter.

4. Identify communication strategies for communicating with children of different age groups.

5. Describe four communication techniques that are useful with children.

6. State the components of a complete health history.

7. Describe two strategies for structural and functional assessment of the family.

8. List three areas that are evaluated as part of nutritional assessment.

III. Review of Essential Concepts

1. The four prerequisites to establish a setting conducive to the interviewing process are:
   a.

   b.

   c.

   d.

2. Various communication strategies are useful when interviewing parents. Identify the purpose of each strategy listed below.
   a. Encouraging the parent to talk—

   b. Directing the focus—

   c. Listening—

d. Silence–

e. Being empathetic–

f. Defining the problem–

g. Solving the problem–

h. Providing anticipatory guidance–

i. Avoiding blocks to communication–

3. List at least 3 signs of information overload.
   a.

   b.

   c.

4. List at least 3 verbal strategies for conducting culturally sensitive interactions.
   a.

   b.

   c.

5. Match the communication strategy to the age group that it is best used with:
   ___ infant
   ___ young child
   ___ school-age child
   ___ adolescent
   a. told what they will do and how they will feel
   b. cuddling
   c. told what is going on and why it is being done
   d. being attentive and not prying

6. Storytelling is a communication strategy in which?
   a. the nurse listens carefully and reflects back the feelings and content of the statements to the client.
   b. books are used in a therapeutic and supportive manner.
   c. the nurse presents statements and has the client fill in the blanks.
   d. the nurse uses the language of the child to probe areas of his thinking.

7. Four nonverbal methods of communication that are utilized with young children are _____, _____, _____, and _____.

8. ___ The objective of each assessment area is the identification of nursing diagnoses. (true or false)

9. The ten major components of a health history for the child and family include:
   a.

   b.

   c.

   d.

   e.

   f.

   g.

   h.

   i.

   j.

10. List the four structural areas of the family assessment that the nurse must consider.
    a.

    b.

    c.

    d.

11. The _____ is a very useful structural assessment tool.

12. ___ The purpose of a nutritional assessment is to evaluate how much weight a child needs to gain. (true or false)

13. A thorough nutritional assessment includes _____, _____, and _____.

14. A method utilized in the clinical examination portion of the nutritional assessment is:

a. fundoscopy
b. arthroscopy
c. anthropometry
d. biopsy

IV. Application, Analysis, and Synthesis of Essential Concepts

A. Experiential Exercise: Interview a preschool child and his family.
  1. It is important to establish a setting for the interview. What is the first thing that should be said to establish this setting?

  2. What blocks to communication may occur during the interview?

  3. What communication techniques are effective in encouraging communication with the child?

  4. Why is it important to include the parents in the problem-solving process?

B. Clinical Situation: Mrs. Fernandez brings her daughter Susan, age 18 months, to the pediatric child clinic for an annual checkup. It is the first time they have visited the clinic. Mrs. Fernandez' English is poor. The Fernandezes have been living in the United States for 6 months.
  1. List at least four verbal strategies that would enhance the cultural sensitivity of the interaction.
    a.

    b.

    c.

    d.

  2. During the interview Mrs. Fernandez focuses her comments on the other four children. How might the nurse redirect the focus of the interview?

  3. What portion of the past-history section of the health history is of particular importance because Susan has been in this country only 6 months?

  4. What information in the family medical history section of the health history should the nurse obtain from Mrs. Fernandez?

  5. In order to assess the family home environment, you would use two tools:
    a.

    b.

C. Clinical Situation: Gwen, age 8, was referred to the nutrition clinic by the nurse practitioner. The nurse was concerned because Gwen's weight was above the 90th percentile for her age. A complete nutritional assessment was performed.
  1. What factors should be included in a dietary history of Gwen?

  2. Identify three methods that Gwen's mother can use to record Gwen's dietary intake.
    a.

    b.

    c.

  3. Anthropometry was performed on Gwen. Why?

  4. What should Gwen be told about the nutritional assessment process?

5. The results of the nutritional assessment revealed that Gwen's mother knows little about nutrition and that Gwen's obesity is the result of her excessive intake of nutrients. Develop two nursing diagnoses based on the assessment results.

a.

b.

V. Suggested Readings

Basch E, and others: Validation of mothers' reports of dietary intake by four to seven year-old children, Am Pub Health 81(11):1314-1317, 1990.

> This study tested the validity of mothers' recall of 46 first-generation Latino immigrant families from the Dominican Republic. The results verified that recall appears to be a useful tool in assessing children's intake of calories and nutrients in this population.

Kristal AR, and others: Development and validation of food use checklist for evaluation of community nutrition interventions, Am Pub Health 80(11):1318-1322, 1990.

> This study reported the development of a new dietary assessment instrument called "Food Behavior Checklist (FBC)," which measures food use related to adopting lower-fat and higher-fiber diets. The FBC is a simplification of the 24-hour recall that consists of 19 simple yes/no questions about foods consumed during the previous day. The instrument was validated on 96 women who were previously administered the 24-hour recall. Agreement between the two instruments was good to excellent on most items. This study provides evidence that a short checklist questionnaire can be employed to assess diet at the group or community level.

Rollins JA: Childhood cancer: siblings draw and tell, Pediatr Nurs 16(1):21-27, 1990.

> As a part of a larger research study of 17 families of children with cancer, 20 healthy siblings, ages 3 to 11 years, were tested using the Kinetic Family Drawing—Revised in one of two oncology clinics in a southwestern state. Data from the drawings and discussions were analyzed to assess psychosocial needs of the siblings. This study confirms that, from the drawings, pediatric nurses can learn a great deal of information left unspoken by the siblings. A comprehensive approach to sibling intervention requires psychosocial assessment of nondisease as well as disease-related stressors. Interventions must then help the families increase their adaptive capacity.

Chapter 7
Physical and Developmental Assessment of the Child

I.   Chapter Overview

Chapter 7 provides the theoretical basis for the performance of a complete pediatric physical assessment and a developmental assessment. Since assessment is the first step in the nursing process, procedures and skills that aid in obtaining accurate and complete data are crucial to students. This chapter provides the base for the performance of a complete physical and developmental assessment in the practicum setting.

II.   Learning Objectives

Upon completion of this chapter, it is expected that the student will be able to:

1.   Prepare a child for a physical examination based on his or her developmental needs.

2.   Perform a physical examination in a sequence appropriate to the child's age.

3.   Recognize expected normal findings for children at various ages.

4.   Record the physical examination according to the head-to-toe format.

5.   Perform a developmental assessment using a standard screening test.

III. Review of Essential Concepts

1.   Five goals that serve as a basis for modifying the normal examination sequence in children are:
a.

b.

c.

d.

e.

2.   List the techniques the nurse might use with an uncooperative child.
a.

b.

c.

d.

e.

f.

g.

3. List the sequence of events in the physical assessment of a child.
   a.

   b.

   c.

   d.

   e.

   f.

   g.

   h.

   i.

   j.

   k.

   l.

   m.

   n.

   o.

   p.

   q.

   r.

   s.

4. In general, children whose growth pattern should be following closely include:
   a. those whose height and weight fall between the 50th and 90th percentile for their age
   b. those whose pattern of growth resembles their parents'
   c. those who fail to show rapid weight gain in the toddler and school-age years
   d. those who show a sudden decrease in a previously steady pattern

5. The best order for taking the vital signs in the infant is _____, _____, and _____.

6. Respirations in the infant are counted _____ because they are irregular.

7. Areas that are assessed in the general appearance section of the physical exam include:
   a. weight
   b. posture
   c. apical pulse
   d. color

8. Match the abnormal color change with its correct definition.
   ___ cyanosis
   ___ erythema
   ___ jaundice
   ___ petechiae
   a. small pinpoint hemorrhages
   b. blue tinge to skin
   c. redness of the skin
   d. yellow staining of the skin

9. What should be recorded when assessing the head of an 8-month-old infant?

10. Criteria that are used when referring a 3-year-old for further evaluation of visual acuity include:
    a. 20/10 vision in both eyes on the Snellen Chart
    b. 20/40 vision in both eyes on the Snellen Chart
    c. 20/30 vision in either eye on the Snellen Chart
    d. 20/50 vision in either eye on the Snellen Chart

11. ___ Respirations in the child older than 8 years are primarily abdominal. (true or false)

12. It is important to record the presence of _____ reflexes if the child is beyond infancy.

13. ___ The Denver Developmental Screening Test (DDST) is composed of four major categories: fine motor-adaptive, cognitive, reflexive, and language. (true or false)

14. The DDST can be used to assess the development of children of ages _____.

15. ___ Delays in the DDST are defined as the failure to perform any item passed by 90% of children of the same age. (true or false)

16. The Denver II differs from the DDST in what respects?

IV. Application, Analysis, and Synthesis of Essential Concepts

A. Clinical Situation: Tia Vang, age 3, is brought to the pediatric clinic for a routine physical exam. Tia has been in this country for 1 year, and Tia's father has been unable to immigrate to this country from Cambodia. Tia's immunizations are up to date. This is Tia's first visit to the clinic.

1. Tia refuses to look at you during the health history interview. What behaviors might indicate her readiness to cooperate during the physical exam and how might you facilitate this process?

2. What method would you use to assess Tia's height?

3. Tia's height and weight are below the 5th percentile for children her age. What additional information should you assess before diagnosing that Tia's growth is not normal?

4. Why would you not want to take Tia's temperature orally?

5. How should Tia's vision be assessed and by what methods?

B. Experiential Exercise: Perform a physical assessment on an infant and a school-age child.

1. What area do you assess after you assess each child's general appearance?

2. How do you obtain each child's height and how is it recorded?

3. By what method do you obtain the heart rate in each child?

4. Data that you obtain when you assess the school-age child's behavior include:

5. You assess the external auditory structures and visualize the internal landmarks of the ear. What did you forget to assess and what method could you use in each of the children?

6. You assess the heart sounds for _____, _____, _____, and _____.

7. The school-age child appears to have an arrhythmia. How do you determine whether this is a sinus arrhythmia?

C. Experiential Exercise: Perform a developmental assessment on a toddler and a preschool child.

1. What do you tell the child's parent before the test is begun?

2. What information do you obtain from the child's parent at the conclusion of the test?

3. How do you determine that a delay is present?

4. How do you score items on the Denver Developmental Screening Test?

5. What should you do if the results of the screening exam are abnormal and the child's mother states that his behavior was typical?

V. Suggested Readings

Castigila PT, Petrina MA: Selecting a developmental screening tool, Pediatr Nurs 11(1):8-16, 1985.

This excellent article explores all aspects of the screening process. The author identifies methods to select tools and addresses the rationale of developmental screening. A review of all developmental tools is provided as well as the sources for obtaining the tools.

Killam PE: Orthopedic assessment of young children: developmental variations, Nurse Pract 14(7):27-36, 1989.

This author discusses three orthopedic variations that may be of concern to parents, but are part of normal development. An under

standing of these common developmental variations in the orthopedic assessment of young children will enable the health care provider to respond to parents' concerns with accurate information and counseling.

Vessey JA, and others: Teaching children about their internal bodies, Pediatr Nurs 16(1):29-33, 1990.

This article discusses appropriate and effective methods, language, and timing for nurses to teach basic anatomy and physiology to early school-age children.

Chapter 8

Health Promotion of the Newborn and Family

I. Chapter Overview

Chapter 8 introduces the nursing considerations of caring for the infant and family, during delivery and in the neonatal period. Profound physiologic and psychologic changes occur as the neonate adjusts to extrauterine life. Students need to be aware of these changes so they can assess the neonate's adaptation and help the parents adjust to family life. At the completion of this chapter the student will know the necessary nursing care for the neonate and his family. This knowledge will enable the student to assess the neonate and his family and to formulate nursing goals and interventions that will promote the normal physiologic and psychologic adjustment and development.

II. Learning Objectives

Upon completion of this chapter, it is expected that the student will be able to:

1. Identify the principal cardio-respiratory changes that occur during transition to extrauterine life.

2. Identify the immature physiologic functioning of each body system and its significance to nursing care of the newborn.

3. Perform an initial and transitional assessment of the newborn based on the Apgar score and periods of reactivity.

4. Perform a newborn physical assessment based on recognition of expected normal findings.

5. Outline a nursing care plan for the newborn in the nursery.

6. Assess and promote parent-infant attachment behavior.

III. Review of Essential Concepts

1. The respiratory changes that occur during the transition to extrauterine life include
_____
_____
_____.

2. ___ A change in the cardiovascular system that occurs after birth involves an increase in pressure on the right side of the heart. (true or false)

3. The most important factor controlling the closure of the ductus arteriosus is:
    a. increased oxygen concentration of the blood
    b. deposition of fibrin and cells
    c. fall of endogenous prostaglandin
    d. presence of metabolic acidosis

4. Factors that predispose the neonate to heat loss include:
    a.

    b.

    c.

5. A limitation of the newborn's gastrointestinal system includes:

a. the inability to digest disaccharides
b. decreased transit time of food passing through the stomach and colon
c. increased storage of glycogen
d. deficiency of the enzyme lipase

6. ___ The kidney of the neonate is unable to concentrate urine. (true or false)
7. The five items that are included in the Apgar score are _____, _____, _____, _____, and _____.
8. The maximum score that an infant can receive on the Apgar is _____.
9. For the first _____ hours the infant is in the first period of reactivity.
10. Behaviors seen during the second period of reactivity include:

11. ___ The state of regular sleep is characterized by closed eyes, irregular breathing, muscle twitching, and reactions to external stimuli. (true or false)
12. ___ The normal head circumference of the neonate is 20 to 21 inches. (true or false)
13. ___ The normal pulse rate of the neonate is 120 to 140 beats/min. (true or false)
14. A reflex that should be present in the normal neonate is:
a. Landau
b. Moro
c. parachute
d. neck-righting
15. Areas to be assessed in the general appearance section of the newborn assessment include:

16. The purpose of assessing the umbilical cord is to determine the presence of _____.
17. Six nursing goals that are the basis for safe and effective care of the neonate are:
a.

b.

c.

d.

e.

f.

18. ___ Vitamin K is administered to the newborn to prevent the occurrence of hemorrhagic disease of the newborn. (true or false)
19. The use of soap is discouraged in the newborn period because it interfaces with _____.
20. Cow's milk is not suitable for the infant's nutrition because it:
a. has too few calories per ounce
b. has too much protein
c. is too dilute
d. has too much calcium
21. ___ The process of the father's attachment to the newborn is called engrossment. (true or false)
22. The reasons that discharge planning and care at home are of increasing importance are that:

23. Common concerns or problems during the period immediately after discharge include:

IV. Application, Analysis, and Synthesis of Essential Concepts

A. Experiential Exercise: Perform an initial and transitional assessment on a newborn based on Apgar score and periods of reactivity.
   1. The five areas you assess to determine the Apgar score include:

   2. The infant received a score of 1 on the heart rate category of the Apgar. This indicates that the neonate's heart rate was _____.
   3. The infant had little difficulty adjusting to extrauterine life. The Apgar score for this infant would be between _____.
   4. What behaviors do you observe to indicate that the infant is in the first period of reactivity?

   5. An appropriate nursing intervention in the first stage of reactivity would include:
   a. performance of initial bath

b. instillation of eye drops before child has contact with the parents

c. allowing mother to breast-feed

d. minimizing contact with parents until temperature has stabilized

B. Experiential Exercise: Determine a neonate's gestational age.

1. Assessment of gestational age is important because:

2. The optimal time for the assessment of gestational age is between _____.

3. The six neuromuscular signs that you assess include:

4. You plot the infant's height, weight, and head circumference on standardized graphs. You determine that the infant is normal for gestational age because:

C. Experiential Exercise: Perform a physical assessment on a newborn.

1. The head circumference of the infant you assess should be between _____. If the head circumference is significantly smaller than the chest circumference, _____ _____.

2. What areas do you assess when you examine the eyes of the neonate?

3. How do you determine that the infant is in the "alert inactivity" behavioral stage?

D. Clinical Situation: Baby Boy Florenz is a 1-day-old infant who is rooming in with his mother. Baby Florenz is a term infant who received a normal newborn examination. He is the first child.

1. Formulate at least three nursing diagnoses for Baby Florenz during the newborn period.

a.

b.

c.

2. List four nursing interventions that should be used to maintain a patent airway in Baby Florenz.

a.

b.

c.

d.

3. What is the rationale for keeping clothes and blankets loose?

4. Why should the administration of silver nitrate or antibiotics to the eyes be delayed 1 hour?

5. What criteria could be utilized to evaluate nursing interventions aimed at maintaining a patent airway in the transition period?

6. What areas should be included in the discharge planning of Baby Florenz and his parents?

E. Clinical Situation: The Cohens have just had their first baby, Sarah. The infant received a normal newborn exam. The Cohens have been attending parenting classes in the hospital and feel comfortable about the routine care of their infant.

1. What behaviors might be assessed to determine if the Cohens have attached to Sarah?

2. Why is it important to know the Cohens' relationship to their own parents?

3. Formulate one nursing diagnosis related to the attachment process.

4. Develop six nursing interventions to facilitate the attachment process.

a.

b.

c.

d.

e.

f.

V.   Suggested Readings

Parker S, Frank D: Jitteriness in full-term neonates: prevalence and correlates, Pediatrics 85(1):17-23, 1990.

The prevalence and correlates of jitteriness were evaluated in a sample of 936 healthy full-term infants. Jitteriness was observed in 44% of this sample. Jittery infants were more likely to be visually inattentive and difficult to console compared with infants who are not jittery. These behaviors adversely affect parent-infant interactions. These findings have important implications for the early parent-infant relationship. Pediatric nurses need to be aware of this problem and be prepared to intervene.

Poland RL, editor: The question of routine neonatal circumcision, New Engl J Med 322(18):1312-1315, 1990.

There is a controversy over the advisability of routine circumcision. The controversy is whether the benefits outweigh the risks. The author cited several recent studies that have linked an increased incidence of urinary tract infection with the uncircumcised male. Some researchers have proposed that circumcision may protect males from infection with the human immunodeficiency virus (HIV). The author concludes that "the risks of circumcision are very small when the procedure is performed by an experienced practitioner." However, the author does not advise routine circumcision.

Porter LS, Sobong LC: Differences in maternal perception of the newborn among adolescents, Pediatr Nurs 16(1):101-104, 1990.

Of the 92 pregnant adolescents who took part in this study, half were placed into a group that participated in a Parenting Enhancement Program (PEP) and the other half were not. Data were collected from all the subjects at five intervals beginning during pregnancy and ending at 3 months postpartum. The purpose of the study was to test the effect of the PEP on adolescent mothers' perceptions of the neonate and to ascertain the extent to which PEP reinforces the effects of maternal age or self-esteem on their perceptions. Results demonstrated some evidence that the PEP was effective in altering the adolescents' perception of their newborn. Further investigation will assist nurses to intervene effectively with adolescent mothers.

Schoen EJ, editor: The status of circumcision of newborns, New Engl Med 322(18):1308-1322, 1990.

The opinion that circumcision prevented cancer of the penis and was associated with lower incidence of cervical cancer in sexual partners was a generally accepted from the 1940s through the 1970s. In the decade of the 70s this belief was questioned and data began to be collected to support or refute this practice. The conclusion of this author is that "the benefits of routine circumcision of newborns as a preventive health measure far exceed the risks of the procedure." The implications for parent counseling are evident.

Chapter 9

Health Problems of the Newborn

I. Chapter Overview

Chapter 9 is concerned with the neonate at high risk for morbidity and mortality because of conditions that are superimposed on the normal course of events associated with birth. Advances in medical technology have improved the survival rate of these compromised neonates. Students must be familiar with the complex care required by the high-risk infant and his family. Effective assessment skills are paramount to successful nursing care of these infants who are at risk. At the completion of this chapter the student will have a foundation for high-risk infant care that can be built upon in the practicum setting..

II. Learning Objectives

Upon completion of this chapter, it is expected that the student will be able to:

1. Recognize common deviations from the normal expectations in the newborn.

2. Perform a systematic assessment of an ill newborn.

3. Outline a general plan of care for a high-risk infant.

4. Discuss the role of the nurse in facilitating positive parent-child relationships.

5. Contrast the characteristics of a premature infant and a full-term infant.

6. Discuss the rationale for screening newborns and for providing genetic counseling for families of a newborn with a hereditary condition.

7. Modify a general care plan to meet the needs of an infant with a specific high-risk health deviation.

III. Review of Essential Concepts

1. Soft-tissue injury usually occurs when there is some degree of disproportion between the _____ and the _____.

2. The most commonly observed scalp lesion is _____, a vaguely outlined area of edematous tissue situated over the portion of the scalp that presents during a vertex delivery.
    a. caput succedaneum
    b. hydrocephalus
    c. cephalhematoma
    d. subdural hematoma

3. Fracture of the _____ is the most common birth injury.

4. Loss of movement on the affected side of the face and an absence of wrinkling of the forehead would be indicative of _____.

5. Nursing care of the neonate with brachial palsy is primarily concerned with _____ of the affected arm.

6. Candidiasis and impetigo are two infections that commonly afflict neonates. Match the following statements with the appropriate infectious process. Mark C if the answer is

candidiasis and I if the answer is impetigo.

a. ____ Candida albicans is the causative organism.

b. ____ Staphylococcus aureus is the causative organism.

c. ____ The infection is characterized by vesicular lesions on untraumatized skin.

d. ____ The infection is characterized by white, curdy patches that cannot be scraped from mucous membranes.

e. ____ The infection frequently follows prolonged antibiotic therapy.

f. ____ The infection is usually treated with systemic and local antibiotics.

7. The high-risk infant may be classified according to:
   a.
   b.
   c.

8. Items to be included in the gastrointestinal assessment of the infant include:

9. Extracellular water content is _____ in a preterm than in a full-term infant.

10. An indication that the preterm infant can breast-feed is:
    a. presence of a rooting reflex
    b. weight of at least 1250 g
    c. presence of a suck reflex
    d. an intolerance to formula

11. Alkaline-base soaps should not be used to clean the skin of the preterm infant because they interfere with the _____ _____.

12. Match the characteristics with type of maturity.
    a. ___ abundant lanugo
    b. ___ presence of subcutaneous fat
    c. ___ cracked skin
      1) premature
      2) postmature
      3) term

13. _____ refers to an increased bilirubin level in the blood.

14. The major clinical manifestation of hyperbilirubinemia is _____.

15. Why do most newborns experience elevated bilirubin levels?

16. A common treatment for hyperbilirubinemia that involves the use of intense fluorescent light is called _____.

17. A factor in the pathophysiology of respiratory distress syndrome is:
    a. decreased pulmonary vascular resistance
    b. failure to establish a functional residual capacity
    c. absence of surfactant
    d. nonreactivity of the baroreceptors

18. ___ The diagnosis of sepsis is always made on the basis of blood cultures. (true or false)

19. Complications of sepsis that the nurse should look for include: _____.

20. Clinical manifestations specific to necrotizing enterocolitis include:

21. A characteristic clinical manifestation of the infant of a diabetic mother not under complete control is:
    a. hyperglycemia
    b. loss of subcutaneous fat
    c. absence of vernix caseosa
    d. largeness for gestational age

22. Drug therapies include administration of

    _____, _____, _____, or _____.

23. A disease spread by ticks is _____ _____.

24. ___ Phenylketonuria (PKU) is inherited as an autosomal-recessive trait. (true or false)

25. The hepatic enzyme, _____ _____, is absent in PKU.

26. The most effective method of identifying neonates with PKU is through _____.

27. ___ Infants with galactosemia usually display notable abnormalities at birth. (true or false)

IV. Application, Analysis, and Synthesis of Essential Concepts

A. Clinical Situation: Baby Boy Jacobs is admitted to the newborn nursery following an uncomplicated vertex delivery. During the initial assessment it is noted that he has a caput succedaneum over the right frontal area.

1. Differentiate between the following types of head trauma that can occur during the birth process.
   a. Caput succedaneum–

   b. Cephalhematoma–

2. Identify the two major nursing goals associated with the care of the neonate with birth-related head trauma.
   a.

   b.

B. Clinical Situation: Care for a high-risk infant.
   1. What is the best method to use in classifying the high-risk infant?

   2. What interventions do you utilize to maintain the thermal stability of the infant?
      a.

      b.

      c.

   3. Why is the prevention of infection such an important goal for the high-risk infant?

   4. The nursing diagnosis for the nursing goal for providing nutrition is:

   5. What assessment parameter could you use to determine if the infant was getting adequate nutrition?

   6. How do you evaluate whether the interventions are successful in preventing skin breakdown?

   7. Four nursing goals developed to prevent an alteration in family process include:
      a.

      b.

      c.

      d.

   8. What is the rationale for encouraging the parents to visit the infant?

C. Experiential Exercise: Care for a neonate who is receiving phototherapy.
   1. What two factors are primarily responsible for the development of physiologic jaundice in the newborn?
      a.

      b.

   2. When would the nurse expect the following phases of physiologic jaundice to occur in the full-term infant?
      a. Onset—

      b. Peak—

      c. Resolution—

   3. Identify the nursing interventions associated with the care of the child receiving phototherapy.
      a.

      b.

      c.

      d.

D. Clinical Situation: Cindy is a premature infant in the ICU. She has recovered from her respiratory distress and has been diagnosed as having an intraventricular hemorrhage. She is suspected of having sepsis.
   1. Postnatally, Cindy may have obtained her infection as a result of:

   2. What are some of the findings that can be observed that suggest sepsis?

   3. The most important nursing goal for Cindy is _____.

E. Clinical Situation: Michael is a premature infant who experienced severe asphyxia at birth. Oral feedings were started within the first 24 hours. He is now having problems with feedings. Necrotizing enterocolitis (NEC) is suspected. He is also anemic.
   1. What factor in Michael's history predisposes him to the development of NEC?

2. The most important nursing responsibility when caring for infants who are at risk for developing NEC is _____.
3. Nursing interventions that would alert the nurse to the presence of NEC include:

F. Clinical Situation: Terry is a 3-day-old infant born to a mother who developed diabetes during pregnancy. Terry was admitted to ICU for observation.
   1. Why is hypoglycemia a common occurrence in infants of diabetic mothers?

   2. Why is feeding begun so early with these infants?

   3. Nursing responsibilities for the infant of a diabetic mother include monitoring the infant for signs of:

V. Suggested Readings

Chasnoff IJ, and others: Cocaine/polydrug use in pregnancy: two-year follow-up, Pediatrics 89(2):284-289, 1992.

> This study of three groups of infants, some of whom were exposed to drugs in utero, found a significant correlation between small head size and developmental scores. Intrauterine exposure to drugs may place infants at risk for developmental outcome, and head growth may be an important biological marker in predicting long-term development in children.

Hayes JS, and others: Managing PKU: an update, MCN 12:119-123, 1987.

> Phenylketonuria is defined and methods of screening for this disorder are reviewed. Management of diet and prevention of infection are primary nursing goals in the care of this disorder. The nursing role is primarily concerned with educating the child, family, and selected community people (teachers, etc.) regarding the screening for and management of children with PKU. A perspective on the pregnant mother who also has PKU is presented.

Ioli JG, Richardson MJ: Giving surfactant to premature infants, Am Nurs, March:59-60, 1990.

> This article discusses the pros and cons of using surfactant replacement therapy to reduce the incident of respiratory distress syndrome.

Rogers MC, editor: Do the right thing: pain relief in infants and children, New Engl Med 326(1):55-56, 1992.

> In this editorial the author comments about a study done by Anand and Hickey that demonstrates the increased risk to neonates who do not receive complete anesthesia during cardiac surgery. The author also raises the general issue of pain relief in neonates and infants in other clinical settings, and contends that it is a professional responsibility to treat pain in neonates and infants as effectively as that of the adult client.

Rose BS: Phototherapy: all wrapped up? Pediatr Nurs 16(1):57-58, 1990.

> This author reports on the advantages of using the Wallaby Phototherapy System (known as the Fiberoptic Blanket). Studies reveal that the "blanket" is as effective as conventional therapy but allows the mother to hold the infant and dispenses with the need for eye protection and control of hypothermia. This therapy will be particularly useful in the home setting.

Rushton CH: Necrotizing enterocolitis, I. Pathogenesis and diagnosis, MCN 15(5):296-300, 1990.

> Although necrotizing enterocolitis is the most common acquired gastrointestinal disease, its etiology and pathology are still controversial. This article thoroughly explores the pathogenesis and diagnosis of this disease. The staging based on clinical manifestations is also presented.

Rushton CH: Necrotizing enterocolitis, II. Treatment and nursing care, MCN 15(5):309-313, 1990.

> This article discusses the role of nurses in assessing and recognizing the signs of NEC. Early detection and treatment can help change the outcome of the more than 20% to 40% of infants with NEC who die. A thorough presentation of the clinical manifestations, surgical treatment, and complications are given. A detailed nursing care summary is the highlight of this article.

Chapter 10

Health Promotion of the Infant and Family

I. Chapter Overview

Chapter 10 explores infancy, the period from birth to 12 months. The focus of this chapter is the normal progression of growth and development and the fostering of optimal health in the infant through anticipatory guidance of the parents. Infancy is the period of the fastest gain in physical size and of the most dramatic developmental achievements of the entire life span. It is characterized by an orderly progression of physical, cognitive, and social maturation, which may be susceptible to positive and negative influences. Upon completion of this chapter the student should have the necessary information base to counsel parents on optimal development.

II. Learning Objectives

Upon completion of this chapter, it is expected that the student will be able to:

1. Identify the major biologic, psychosocial, cognitive, and social developments of the first year.

2. Relate parent-child attachment, separation anxiety, and stranger fear to developmental achievements during infancy.

3. Provide anticipatory guidance to parents regarding common parental concerns during infancy.

4. Provide parents with feeding recommendations for infants.

5. Outline immunization requirements during infancy.

6. List the general contraindications, precautions, and administration routes for immunizations.

7. Provide anticipatory guidance to parents regarding injury prevention based on the infant's developmental achievements.

III. Review of Essential Concepts

1. An infant who is 5 months of age should have _____ his birth weight.
2. Binocularity should be well established by the age of _____.
3. A physiologic characteristic of a 5-month-old is:
    a. the present of iron deficiency anemia
    b. presence of drooling
    c. eruption of the first tooth
    d. adult level of fat absorption
4. List two reasons why infants are susceptible to dehydration.
    a.

    b.

5. The fine motor development of a 3-month-old can best be described by:
    a. the ability to transfer objects
    b. the desire to grasp an object
    c. the ability to voluntarily grasp an object
    d. the presence of a pincer grasp

6. The gross motor development of a 6-month-old can best be described by:
   a. the ability to roll from back to abdomen
   b. the ability to sit unsupported
   c. the ability to crawl
   d. the ability to pull self to standing position
7. ___ The infant is in Erikson's stage of development. (true or false)
8. Piaget's stage of secondary circular reactions is characterized by:
   a. totally autistic behavior
   b. recognizing familiar behavior
   c. attainment of object permanence
   d. becoming bored when left alone
9. The two components of cognitive development that are necessary for attachment are:
   a.

   b.

10. ___ At 3 months, the infant displays a definite preference for the mother. (true or false)
11. Stranger anxiety is defined as:

12. An 8-month-old infant's language ability can best be described as:
   a. the ability to say dada
   b. the ability to understand no
   c. the ability to say mama
   d. the ability to respond to own name
13. Stimulation (in the form of play) is as important for _____ growth as food is for biologic growth.
14. Appropriate toys for a 4-month-old child are:

15. How should the parents of a temperamentally active child modify their childrearing practices?

16. ___ Problems with dental development are associated with the use of a pacifier. (true or false)
17. A quick guide to assessment of deciduous teeth during the first year is _____ _____.

18. The main reason for shoes when the ch has started walking is for _____
19. Human milk is deficient in the mine _____ and supplements of _____ per day should be given.
20. ___ The amount of formula that a 6-mon old should be taking at each of five feedi is 8 oz. (true or false)
21. List the reasons why it is not advisable introduce solid foods to a 3-month-infant.
   a.

   b.

   c.

   d.

22. The first solid that is introduced _____ because of its high _____ content.
23. ___ Each new solid food is introduced al for 4 to 7 days to detect food allergies. (t or false)
24. The management of night crying includes
   a. putting child in own bed while awake
   b. arranging a separate sleeping area
   c. placing child in parents' bed for comfor
   d. rocking child until asleep
25. ___ During infancy teeth are cleaned wit soft toothbrush. (true or false)
26. A 7-month-old's immunization record sho read:
   a. DTP at 2, 4 months; TOPV at 2, 4 mont
   b. DTP at 2, 4 months; TOPV at 2, 4 months; HbCV at 2, 6 months
   c. DTP at 2, 4, 6 months; TOPV at 2 months; HbCV at 2, 4, 6 months; HBV birth, 2 months, possibly 6 months
   d. DTP at 2 months; TOPV at 2, 4, 6 mont
27. Common reactions to a DTP immunizat include:

28. A contraindication for all immunizations
   a. an upper respiratory infection
   b. antibiotic therapy
   c. steroid therapy
   d. gastritis
29. The leading cause of fatal injury in child under 1 year of age is _____
30. Guidelines to prevent accidental injuries a 2-month-old child include:
   a. teaching child to swim to prevent drown
   b. using a pillow to prevent aspiration

c. using warm mist vaporizer to prevent chilling

d. shaking baby powder on own hands first to prevent choking

IV. Application, Analysis, and Synthesis of Essential Concepts

A. Clinical Situation: Mrs. Backer brings 7-month-old Jerry to the well-child clinic for his checkup. During the course of the examination Mrs. Backer says that Jerry is teething, has shown little interest in breast-feeding, and cries when she leaves the room. She has been reading Parents magazine and is concerned that Jerry is not "doing" what the magazine states he should be "doing."

1. Jerry was 7 pounds at birth. At this visit he weighs 16 pounds. Is this weight normal for his age?

2. What fine motor, gross motor, language, and social developmental milestones does the nurse assess in Jerry that lead to a determination that Jerry is developing normally?

3. What nursing intervention might you suggest to Mrs. Backer regarding Jerry's crying when she leaves the room?

4. List the interventions that Mrs. Backer could implement to relieve teething pain.
   a.

   b.

5. What might Jerry's lack of interest in breast-feeding indicate, and what intervention should you suggest to Jerry's mother?

6. List the interventions that Mrs. Backer can use to promote good dental health in Jerry.
   a.

   b.

   c.

   d.

   e.

B. Clinical Situation: Rachel is a 4-month-old infant who is at the clinic for her checkup. Rachel's mother states that she is having difficulty managing Rachel because nothing she tries works twice, and she is concerned about Rachel's sleeping pattern.

1. What behaviors are assessed to determine whether Rachel is in Piaget's stage of secondary circular reactions?

2. What should the nurse assess regarding Rachel's sleeping pattern?
   a.

   b.

   c.

   d.

   e.

3. Rachel's mother will start Rachel on solid foods before the next checkup. What guidelines should be given to her?
   a.

   b.

   c.

   d.

   e.

   f.

   g.

C. Experiential Exercise: Administer immunizations to an infant.
   1. What factors do you need to assess in the

infant that might prevent you from administering immunizations?

2. What two nursing interventions should be utilized to properly administer immunizations?
   a.

   b.

3. What is the safest site for administration of immunizations in the infant?

4. What are the nursing interventions associated with a DTP vaccine administration?
   a.

   b.

   c.

   d.

D. Experiential Exercises: Teach the parents of an infant who is 8 to 12 months old how to prevent accidental injury to their child.
   1. What developmental landmarks do you assess in the infant that predispose him to injury?

   2. What interventions might you suggest to prevent burns in the child?
      a.

      b.

      c.

      d.

      e.

3. What is the rationale for keeping the bathroom door closed?

4. Why is choking still such a problem in this age group?

5. What is the rationale for not administering medications as candy?

6. The parents inform you that their infant frequently spends time at the grandparents' home. What nursing intervention should you suggest to them?

V. Suggested Readings

Balameyer B: Sleep disturbances of the infant and toddler, Pediatr Nurs 16(5):447-452, 1990.

> The physiology of sleep and sleep states in children are presented. Two common sleep disorders in infants and toddlers—sleeplessness and arousal disorders—are discussed. Nursing assessment parameters and interventions that can effectively reduce sleep disorders are offered.

Griffin MT, and others: Risk of seizure and encephalopathy after immunization with the Diphtheria-Pertussis vaccine, JAMA 263(12):1641-1645, 1990.

> The authors evaluated 38,171 children in Tennessee who received DTP immunizations in their first 3 years of life. The authors found no evidence that in the 0-3 days after the immunization the risk of afebrile seizures or acute asymptomatic seizures was not increased. The risk of febrile seizures was slightly increased following DPT immunization.

Snow LS, Fry MT: Formula feeding in the first year of life, Pediatr Nurs 16(5):442-446, 1990.

> By 2 months of age, 60% of all infants in the United States are completely formula fed. Nursing diagnosis and assessment provide the framework for discussing the following issues: (1) what to feed infants, (2) how to evaluate nutritional intake and feeding problems, (3) safety considerations, and (4) the social aspects of feeding. A useful guide for nurses to educate and support parents of formula-fed infants.

Chapter 11
Health Problems During Infancy

I. Chapter Overview

Chapter 11 introduces common health problems of the first year of life. They are usually influenced by environmental factors affecting the physical or psychologic development of the child due to the infant's immature physiologic system. Some have no "etiology." Students need to be aware of these health problems because most of them are amenable to prevention, and prompt identification and treatment will avert problems later in life. At the completion of this chapter the student should have the foundation to provide nursing care to children with these health problems and their families.

II. Learning Objectives

Upon completion of this chapter, it is expected that the student will be able to:

1. Identify children at increased risk for developing nutritional disturbances.

2. Outline a nutritional counseling plan for vitamin or mineral deficiency and excess.

3. Outline a dietary plan for parents when the infant is sensitive to milk.

4. List measures that can be used to alleviate colic.

5. Plan nursing care that meets the physical and emotional needs of the nonorganic failure-to-thrive child and parent.

6. Provide nursing care that meets the immediate and long-term needs of the family who has lost a child from sudden infant death syndrome.

7. Identify the stresses and needs of the family whose child is being monitored at home for apnea.

8. Identify characteristics of children with autism.

III. Review of Essential Concepts

1. ___ Vitamin D is necessary for the absorption of calcium and phosphorus in the body. (true or false)
2. Vitamin excess is often a result of
_____.
3. The deficiency of Vitamin C is referred to as:
    a. rickets
    b. scurvy
    c. pellagra
    d. beriberi
4. ___ Excess sodium in the diet may lead to the development of hypotension. (true or false)
5. The clinical manifestations of a zinc deficiency include:

6. Sources of iron in the diet include:

7. The American Academy of Pediatrics recommends that fat in the diet should not be limited in children _____ _____ years, and in youngsters older than _____, fat should provide _____ to _____ of calories.

8. Kwashiorkor is defined as:
   a. deficiency of calories
   b. deficiency of calories and protein
   c. deficiency of fats and carbohydrates
   d. deficiency of protein with adequate calories

9. The diagnosis of cow's milk intolerance is initially made _____.

10. Lactose intolerance involves deficiency of the enzyme _____.

11. Manifestations of lactose intolerance are:

12. Match the feeding problem with its definition.
   ___ regurgitation
   ___ spitting up
   ___ colic
   ___ rumination
   a. paroxysmal abdominal pain
   b. voluntary return of food into the mouth
   c. return of undigested food from the stomach
   d. dribbling of unswallowed formula

13. List the elements of the nursing assessment that would be noted regarding colic.
   a.
   b.
   c.
   d.
   e.
   f.
   g.

14. ___ Rumination is usually considered to be the result of disturbed parent-child relationship. (true or false)

15. The primary objective in the nursing care of the child who is ruminating is:

16. ___ A characteristic of children who fail to thrive is their intense interest in social interaction. (true or false)

17. Parents of the failure-to-thrive infant are usually:

18. The most important nursing goal for the failure-to-thrive infant is _____.

19. List the guidelines that should be utilized for the feeding interaction of the failure-to-thrive infant.
   a.
   b.
   c.
   d.
   e.
   f.
   g.

20. The four groups of children who are considered at risk for sudden infant death syndrome (SIDS) are:
   a.
   b.
   c.
   d.

21. One approach to the nursing care for families of SIDS infants is based on:

22. One of the most important aspects of the care of the parents following a SIDS death is:

23. The most widely used test in the diagnostic evaluation of apnea of infancy is the _____.

24. The therapeutic management of the infant with apnea involves the use of _____ and _____ drugs.

25. Three safety measures that should be discussed with parents of the infant being monitored at home are:
   a.
   b.
   c.

26. A predominant characteristic of infantile autism is:
  a. abnormal concern for varied stimulation
  b. presence of stranger anxiety at an early age
  c. extreme interpersonal isolation
  d. social advancement that stops at 7-month level

IV. Application, Analysis, and Synthesis of Essential Concepts

A. Clinical Situation: Mr. Bacon brings his 10-month-old into the pediatric clinic for the well-child visit. Upon examination it is noted that the child's weight gain has leveled off and he exhibits signs of a niacin deficiency. The Bacons belong to the Seventh Day Adventist faith.
  1. What risk factors should the nurse have assessed in previous well-child visits that might have prevented the nutritional problems?

  2. It is important that during the nutritional assessment of the Bacon's infant that the nurse assess _____.
  3. List the items that would be included as interventions to help alleviate the nutritional problems of the Bacons' infant:
    a.

    b.

    c.

    d.

    e.

    f.

  4. How would you evaluate whether your interventions were successful in treating the nutritional problem?

B. Experiential Exercise: Care for a child who has nonorganic failure to thrive and his family.

  1. Identify three nursing goals for the nursing diagnosis of potential for trauma, neglect.
    a.

    b.

    c.

  2. What characteristics did you assess in the infant that are indicative of failure-to-thrive infants?

  3. To evaluate whether the interventions have been successful in alleviating the nutritional problem, you would evaluate whether:

  4. Develop one nursing diagnosis that could be used when working with the parents.

C. Clinical Situation: Mr. and Mrs. Cohen arrive in the Emergency Room with their infant. The Cohens discovered that their infant had stopped breathing and called the rescue team, but the child could not be resuscitated.
  1. List the interventions that should be used to support the parents on the discovery of the infant.
    a.

    b.

    c.

  2. In addition to supporting the parents, another nursing goal to meet the immediate needs of the family who have lost a child from SIDS is _____.
  3. What intervention could be used to help the parents adjust to the loss?
    a.

    b.

    c.

D. Clinical Situation: Tommy, a 1-month-old infant, is admitted to the hospital for a diagnostic workup for apnea of infancy. Tommy's parents called the pediatrician when they noticed that Tommy had periods where he stopped breathing and turned "blue."

1. Nursing interventions aimed at supporting the parents of the infant with infantile apnea are:

2. Why is safety a major area of nursing intervention if the infant is to be monitored at home?

3. What is the rationale for informing the local utility and rescue squad of the home monitoring?

4. To lessen the continuous responsibility of monitoring for the parents, nursing interventions should be aimed at:

5. Tommy's mother informs the nurse that he vomits small amounts of formula after he feeds. How can the nurse distinguish between vomiting and spitting up?

E. Experiential Exercise: Care for a child with infantile autism.
   1. The child's intellectual functioning is assessed. The majority of autistic children _____.

   2. The goals used in the management of autism include:

V. Suggested Readings

Carey WB, editor: Colic: exasperating but fascinating and gratifying, Pediatrics 84(3):568-569, 1989.

   The author critically reviews a study done by Barr and associates on colic and infant temperament. Three other studies are also reviewed, and interventions with the parents are presented.

Chesney RW: Requirements and upper limits of vitamin D intake in the term neonate, infant and older child, Pediatr 116(2):159-165, 1990.

   This review attempts to define the upper limits of vitamin D intake that will prevent vitamin D deficiency, will avoid toxic effects, and at the same time will be safe.

Poland RL, editor: Vitamin E for prevention of perinatal intracranial hemorrhage, Pediatrics 85(5):865-867, 1990.

   This author did a preliminary review of the research concerning vitamin E and prevention of intracranial hemorrhage. The resulting evidence suggests that vitamin E may have a role in the prevention of intracranial hemorrhage in the smallest premature neonates.

Chapter 12

Health Promotion of the Toddler and Family

I.   Chapter Overview

Chapter 12 presents the issues relevant to the toddler period of development. Since this is a time of accelerated psychosocial, cognitive, and adaptive changes, students need to be aware of behavior problems that may occur. At the completion of this chapter, the student will understand the toddler's needs and be aware of areas of special concern to parents. This knowledge enables the student to develop nursing goals and interventions that provide support for the normal development of the toddler and help parents cope with the associated developmental difficulties.

II. Learning Objectives

Upon completion of this chapter, it is expected that the student will be able to:

1.   Identify the major biologic, psychosocial, cognitive, and social developments during the toddler years.

2.   Relate separation anxiety and negativism to developmental tasks.

3.   Recognize readiness for toilet training and offer parents guidelines.

4.   Prepare toddlers for the birth of a sibling.

5.   Provide parents with guidelines for handling temper tantrums.

6.   Provide parents with feeding recommendations.

7.   Outline a preventive dental hygiene plan for toddlers.

8.   Provide anticipatory guidance to parents regarding injury prevention based on the toddler's developmental achievements.

III. Review of Essential Concepts

1.   The toddler period is the time between _____ and _____.

2.   The growth rate slows considerably during the toddler years, and the birth weight is quadrupled by _____ years of age.

3.   ___ When plotted on height and weight graphs, the toddler's growth curve is usually a steady, upward curve, which is steplike in nature. (true or false)

4.   Why does the toddler exhibit a squat, potbellied appearance?

5.   Visual acuity of _____ is achieved during the toddler years, although _____ is considered acceptable.

6.   One of the most prominent changes in the gastrointestinal system is the voluntary control of _____.

7.   The major gross motor skill acquired during the toddler years is _____.

8. Identify the seven major psychosocial developmental tasks that must be dealt with during the toddler years.

a.

b.

c.

d.

e.

f.

g.

9. According to Erikson, the developmental task of toddlerhood is acquiring a sense of _____ while overcoming a sense of _____ and _____.

10. Identify two characteristics that are typical of toddlers in their quest for autonomy.

a.
b.

11. According to Erickson, the development of ego is evident when the child is able to _____.

12. A child of 21 months would be expected to be in Piaget's stage of:

a. tertiary circular reactions
b. preoperations
c. coordination of secondary schemata and their application to new situations
d. secondary circular reactions
e. invention of new means through mental combinations

13. At approximately 2 years of age the child enters the _____ of cognitive development.

14. A toddler's reasoning can best be described as being:

a. transductive
b. inductive
c. deductive

15. Match the following terms related to toddler behavior with their definitions.

a. ___ transductive reasoning
b. ___ centration
c. ___ ritualism
d. ___ animism
e. ___ negativism

1) the need to maintain sameness and reliability
2) thinking that progresses from the particular to the general

3) the tendency to focus on one aspect rather than considering all possible alternatives
4) persistent negative response to requests
5) attribution of lifelike qualities to inanimate objects

16. ___ The development of body image closely parallels cognitive development. (true or false)

17. Briefly describe the two phases of the toddler's task of differentiation of self from significant others.

a. Separation—

b. Individuation—

18. ___ The most striking feature of language development in the toddler is the number of new vocabulary words acquired. (true or false)

19. The typical child of 2 years has a vocabulary of approximately _____ words, and approximately _____ percent of this speech is understandable.

20. In the realm of personal-social behavior, the toddler's developing skills of _____ are evident in all areas.

21. The child of 2 years can be expected to:

a. use expressive jargon
b. build a tower of 8 cubes
c. have a vocabulary of 500 words
d. run fairly well with wide stance

22. The solitary play of infancy progresses to _____ play in the toddler.

23. In terms of growth and development, the age of _____ is a particularly integrated period of developmental achievement.

24. Physical and psychological readiness for toilet training is not completed until the _____.

25. ___ Bowel training is usually accomplished before bladder training in the toddler. (true or false)

26. Sibling rivalry seems to be most pronounced in the _____ child.

27. ___ It is advisable to prepare the toddler for the birth of a sibling at least 6 months in advance. (true or false)

28. A particular form of discipline that is well suited to the physical needs and cognitive understanding of this age child is _____.

29. Temper tantrums are a means by which toddlers assert their _____.
30. One method by which a parent can deal with negativism is be reducing _____.
31. The decreased nutritional requirements of the toddler are manifested in a phenomenon known as _____.
32. A good rule of thumb in determining the appropriate serving size for a toddler is to give _____ of food for each year of age.
33. The toddler should see a dentist after the first teeth erupt and no later than the age of _____ years, when primary dentition is completed.
34. The most effective methods for plaque removal are _____ and _____.
35. When adequate amounts of _____ are ingested, the incidence of tooth decay _____.
36. ___ is a statement that accurately describes nursing-bottle caries.
    a. Nursing-bottle caries occurs in children between 8 and 18 months of age.
    b. The syndrome is distinguished by protruding upper front teeth resulting from sucking on a hard nipple.
    c. The syndrome does not occur when the child has been breast fed.
    d. Giving a bottle of milk at nap or bedtime predisposes the child to this syndrome.
37. _____ cause more deaths in children 1 to 4 years of age than in any other childhood period except adolescence.
38. What is the implication of the previous statement?

39. Briefly describe the Rule of Fours that applies to the use of car restraint systems.

40. _____ are the most common type of thermal injury in children.
41. The major reason for accidental poisoning in young children is _____.

IV. Application, Analysis, and Synthesis of Essential Concepts

A. Clinical Situation: A young mother brings her 2-year-old son, David, into a well-child clinic for a routine checkup. The child is apprehensive and clings to his mother. Height and weight are obtained; the child's height is 35 in (89 cm) and his weight is 30 lb (13.64 kg).

1. Plot David's height and weight on a growth chart. How do his measurements compare to the norms for this age?
   a. Height–

   b. Weight–

2. David's mother is concerned because he has gained only 2 pounds and grown 2 inches since his 18-month checkup. What information should be provided to his mother regarding toddler growth patterns?

3. Identify three developmental milestones that David should have accomplished in the following areas.
   a. Gross motor development–

   b. Fine motor development–

   c. Language development–

4. David's mother states that when he is with other children of his age, he plays near them but makes no attempt to interact with them. What information regarding the toddler's play habits should be provided?

5. What information should be provided to David's mother regarding the selection of appropriate play activities?
   a.

   b.

   c.

6. David is not yet toilet trained. His mother asks when she should begin trying to train

him. The nurse's most appropriate response
should be:

a. David will need to be able to sit on the
toilet for 10 to 15 minutes at a time.

b. A factor in successful training is the
child's desire to please the mother by controlling impulses to defecate and urinate.

c. Bladder training should be attempted
first since the child usually has a stronger
and more regular urge to urinate.

d. Attempts to begin toilet training before age
3 are usually unsuccessful because myelin-
ization of the spinal cord is incomplete.

7. David's mother asks questions about dental
care. List four components for a preventive
dental hygiene plan for a toddler.

a.

b.

c.

d.

B. Experiential Exercise: Interview the parents of
a toddler about negativism, management of
temper tantrums, methods of discipline, and
eating and sleep patterns. Answer the following questions and include specific responses
that illustrate these concepts.

1. How is negativism most often manifested in
the toddler?

2. The most effective method of dealing with
negativism is to reduce the opportunity for a
_____.

3. How does negativism contribute to the toddler's acquisition of a sense of autonomy?

4. Why are temper tantrums so prevalent in
the toddler age group?

5. Why does physiologic anorexia occur in the
toddler?

6. Identify four eating behaviors that are characteristic of the toddler.

a.

b.

c.

d.

7. Why is nutritional counseling for parents with
toddlers an important nursing intervention?

8. Sleep problems are common in this age
group. The problems are probably related to
_____ .

9. What are two interventions a parent can
use to reduce sleep problems?

a.

b.

C. Experiential Exercise: Assess the home of a
toddler for the presence of potential safety
hazards. Answer the following questions and
include specific examples that illustrate
these concepts.

1. Identify the two key determinants in injury
prevention.

a.

b.

2. Why is there a critical increase in injuries
during the toddler years?

3. What categories of injuries are common during the toddler years?

a.

b.

c.

d.

e.

f.

g.

4. Identify at least five factors in the home that
could pose a safety hazard to the toddler.

a.

b.

c.

d.

e.

5. Match the following developmental accomplishments with the appropriate safety measures. Answers may be used more than once.
   a. ___walks, runs, climbs
   b. ___ exhibits curiosity
   c. ___ pulls objects
   d. ___ puts things in mouth
      a. Closely supervise when near a source of water.
      b. Choose toys without removable parts.
      c. Turn pot handles toward back of stove.
      d. Place all toxic agents out of reach in a locked cabinet.
      e. Place child-protector caps on all medicines and poisons.
      f. Cover electrical outlets with protective plastic caps.
      g. Avoid giving sharp or pointed objects.
      h. Keep tablecloth out of child's reach.
      i. Lock fences and doors if not directly supervising children.

6. _____
   cause more accidental deaths after the age of 1 year than any other type of injury. What intervention can parents employ to reduce the majority of injuries?

V. Suggested Readings

Committee on Accident and Poison Prevention: Ride-on mower injuries in children, Am Pediatrics, 1990.

> The authors discuss prevention of injury, parent education, operating age and training requirements, and product information and safety devices. Parent education is essential to the prevention of these injuries.

Honig, JC: Preparing preschool-aged children to be siblings, Am J Maternal Child Nurs 11(1):37-43, 1986.

> In this selection, the reactions of young children to the birth of a sibling are examined. This provides a framework for a program for siblings-to-be that is designed to help children cope with the birth of a sibling. A complete curriculum and annotated bibliography supplement the description of one successful sibling preparation program.

Stadtler AC: Preventing encopresis, Pediatr Nurs 15(3):282-284, 1989.

> This article explores the problem of encopresis. The role of the nurse in providing anticipatory guidance and education to help prevent this condition is explored. The article emphasizes the importance of the nurses' preventive role, which can significantly alter the outcome of this disorder.

Chapter 13

Health Promotion of the Preschooler and Family

I.   Chapter Overview

Chapter 13 focuses on the development of the child in the preschool period, which spans the ages of 3 to 5 years. Since this period completes what is considered to be the most critical period of emotional and psychologic development, students need to be aware of some of the issues for this age group. Upon completion of the chapter, the student will have a knowledge of the preschooler's needs and be aware of the areas that are of special concern to parents. This knowledge will enable the student to develop nursing goals and interventions that provide support for the normal development of the preschooler and assist parents in coping with associated developmental difficulties.

II.   Learning Objectives

Upon completion of this chapter, it is expected that the student will be able to:

1.   Identify the major biologic, psychosocial, cognitive, moral, spiritual, and social developments that occur during the preschool years.

2.   List the benefits of imaginary playmates.

3.   Prepare preschoolers for nursery or daycare experience.

4.   Provide parents with guidelines for sex education.

5.   Provide parents with guidelines for dealing with the child's fears and sleep problems.

6.   Recognize the causes of stuttering during the preschool years.

7.   Offer parents suggestions for preventing speech problems.

8.   Recognize feeding patterns of preschoolers.

9.   Provide parents anticipatory guidance regarding injury prevention based on the preschooler's developmental achievements.

III. Review of Essential Concepts

1.   The preschool years, a period from _____ years of age to the completion of the _____ year, comprises the end of early childhood.

2.   During the preschool years, physical growth continues to _____ and _____.

3.   A great deal of learning takes place during the preschool years. Identify three types of knowledge that are attained during this period.
    a.

    b.

    c.

4. According to Erikson, the chief psychosocial task of the preschool period is acquiring a sense of _____.

5. A major task for preschoolers is the development of the _____ or _____.

6. One of the tasks related to the preschool period is _____ for school and _____.

7. The two stages that comprise Piaget's pre-operational phase are:
   a.

   b.

8. Identify one of the major transitions that occurs during the preoperational stage of development.

9. _____ continues to develop during the preschool period. _____ remains primarily a vehicle of _____ communication.

10. _____ resembles logical thought.

11. Preschoolers' thinking is often described as _____, since they believe that thoughts are all-powerful.

12. ___ Preschoolers have poorly defined body boundaries and little knowledge of their internal anatomy. (true or false)

13. List two examples that demonstrate that the preschool child has relinquished much of the stranger anxiety and fear of separation of earlier years.
    a.

    b.

14. ___ During the preschool years, vocabulary increases dramatically. (true or false)

15. _____ speech is a common characteristic during the early preschool years.

16. The typical child of 5 years can be expected to have a vocabulary consisting of at least _____ words.

17. How does the preschooler differ from the toddler in demonstrating a sense of autonomy?
    a.

    b.

18. The type of play that is most apparent during the preschool years is _____ play.

19. The appearance of imaginary playmates usually occurs between the ages of _____ and _____ years.

20. Identify three functions that are served by imaginary playmates.
    a.

    b.

    c.

21. The child of 4 years of age can be expected to:
    a. walk down stairs using alternate footing
    b. tie shoelaces
    c. use sentences of 6 to 8 words
    d. question what parents think

22. List three opportunities that nursery schools and daycare centers provide for children.
    a.

    b.

    c.

23. What factors should parents consider when choosing a preschool or daycare program?
    a.

    b.

    c.

    d.

    e.

    f.

    g.

    h.

    i.

    j.

24. In terms of overall evaluation of a program, the most important factor is _____ _____of the facility.

25. List the two rules that govern answering a child's questions about sex or other sensitive issues.
    a.

    b.

26. _____ in the preschool child is a normal part of sexual curiosity and exploration.

27. The most critical period for speech development occurs between _____ and _____ years of age.

28. Why is stuttering a common occurrence during the preschool years?

29. Identify some of the child's most common fears during the preschool years.
   a.

   b.

   c.

   d.

   e.

   f.

30. Identify the most effective ways to help children overcome their fears.

31. The _____ is an excellent tool to assess articulation skills in the child.

32. Nutritional requirements for preschoolers are similar to those for _____.
   _____ years of age is a period from the resurgence of finicky eating.
   The child of _____ is influenced by the food habits of others and is ready for the social side of eating.

33. What fact should be stressed to parents of preschoolers in the course of nutritional counseling?

34. Identify five reasons why preschool children are subject to sleep problems.
   a.

   b.

   c.

   d.

   e.

35. Why is dental care essential for the preschool child?

   a.

   b.

36. ___ During the preschool years, the emphasis on injury prevention is placed on education for safety and potential hazards. (true or false)

IV. Application, Analysis, and Synthesis of Essential Concepts

A. Clinical Situation: Frank Squire, who will be 5 years old next month, is brought to the pediatrician's office by his mother for a well-child visit. Height and weight are obtained. The child's height is 42 in. (106.6 cm), and his weight is 39 lbs (17.69 kg).

1. Plot Frank's height and weight on a growth chart. How do his measurements compare with the norms for this age?
   a. Height–

   b. Weight–

2. What information could be given to Frank's mother regarding the physical growth of the preschooler?

3. Before the physical examination, the nurse questions Mrs. Squire about Frank's developmental progress. Identify three developmental milestones that Frank should have accomplished in the following areas.
   a. Gross motor development–

   b. Fine motor development–

   c. Language development–

4. Mrs. Squire says that Frank spends most of his time playing with his imaginary friend, Oscar. She wonders if this phase will pass. What information should be given to her?

5. Mrs. Squire states that Frank has several toys but only plays with a few. What types of playthings and activities could be recommended to foster Frank's development?

a. Physical play–

b. Dramatic play–

c. Creative play–

d. Quiet play–

6. Mrs. Squire is very concerned about child safety. What developmental achievements make Frank more prone to injury?

B. Experiential Exercise: Interview the parents of a child who attends a preschool program. Answer the following questions and include specific responses to illustrate these concepts.

1. What is the most important aspect of a preschool or daycare program?

2. What specific factors should be considered when selecting a preschool program?

a.

b.

c.

d.

e.

f.

g.

h.

i.

j.

3. What should parents do when visiting a facility they are considering for their child?

a.

b.

c.

d.

4. How should parents prepare the child for the preschool experience?

a.

b.

c.

d.

C. Experiential Exercise: Interview the parents of a preschool child about the following common parental concerns: sex education, sleep disturbances, and eating patterns. Answer the following questions and include specific responses to illustrate these concepts.

1. Why is the preschool stage of development appropriate for beginning sex education?

2. What two mistakes should parents avoid when answering their children's questions about sex?

a.

b.

3. Identify the rationales for each of the following interventions that promote the sex education of the preschool child.

a. Determining what the child thinks–

b. Being honest–

4. What sleep problems occur in this age group that might concern parents?

5. What interventions could be suggested to parents to deal with this problem?
   a.

   b.

   c.

   d.

6. What is the primary concern of parents regarding the preschool child's diet?

7. Describe one intervention that might decrease this parental concern.

V. Suggested Readings

Aquilino ML, Ely J: Parents and the sexuality of preschool children, Pediatr Nurs 11(1):41-46, 1985.

> This article reports on a survey of 81 parents of preschool children about the sexual activity and curiosity of 3- to 5-year-olds. It was determined that most of the parents were knowledgeable and responded positively to situations involving normal preschool sexual activities but that their comfort with childhood sexuality varied. The implications for presenting information to parents about childhood sexuality are presented.

Edgil A, Wood K, Smith D: Sleep problems of older infants and preschool children, Pediatr Nurs 11(2):87-89, 1985.

> This article examines current knowledge about the various early childhood sleep disturbances that are sources of major concern to parents. It then focuses on a study designed to identify sleep behaviors described by mothers as problems, sleep goals that mothers have for their children, family consequences of children's sleep problems, various systems involved in promoting or preventing sleep problems, and environmental factors related to sleep problems. The findings, their significance to nursing practice, and implications for future research are described in detail.

Summers KH: Establishment of a hospital-based children's sick room, Pediatr Nurs 14(1):38-39, 1988.

> The author discusses a hospital-based child care program called "Children's Sick Room." This program offers affordable care to children who are not quite ready to appear at child-care facilities but would benefit from temporary care.

Chapter 14

Health Problems of Early Childhood

I. Chapter Overview

Chapter 14 introduces nursing considerations essential to the care of the young child experiencing health problems. Although many of these problems can be effectively managed in the home environment, students need to be aware that a potential exists for long-term consequences if appropriate interventions are not instituted promptly. At the completion of this chapter, the student will have a knowledge of commonly encountered health problems of early childhood. This knowledge will enable the student to develop nursing goals and interventions directed at returning the child and family to a state of optimum health.

II. Learning Objectives

Upon completion of this chapter, it is expected that the student will be able to:

1. Describe the major characteristics of communicable diseases of childhood.

2. List three principles of nursing care of children with communicable diseases.

3. Distinguish between aphthous stomatitis and herpetic gingivostomatitis.

4. Outline a teaching plan designed to prevent transmission of intestinal parasites.

5. Identify the principles in the emergency treatment of poisoning.

6. Describe the nursing care of the child with lead poisoning.

7. State three factors thought to be associated with child abuse.

8. State four areas of the history that should arouse suspicion of abuse.

9. Describe the nursing care of the abused child.

III. Review of Essential Concepts

1. Identify four factors that are helpful in identifying communicable diseases in children.
    a.

    b.

    c.

    d.

2. List the four nursing goals in the care of the child and family with a communicable disease.
    a.

    b.

    c.

    d.

3. Primary prevention of communicable disease rests almost exclusively on _____ _____.

4. Nursing interventions to prevent the spread of communicable disease include:
  a.

  b.

5. List the three groups of children who are at risk for developing serious or fatal complications from communicable diseases.
  a.

  b.

  c.

6. List some measures to relieve the itching of skin rashes caused by a communicable disease.
  a.

  b.

  c.

  d.

  e.

7. Define conjunctivitis.

8. Identify the most common causes of conjunctivitis in the following groups.
  a. Recurrent conjunctivitis in infants—

  b. Acute conjunctivitis in children—

9. The distinguishing symptom of bacterial conjunctivitis is _____.

10. ____ Viral conjunctivitis usually occurs in association with an upper respiratory infection. (true or false)

11. ____ The primary sign of conjunctivitis caused by a foreign body is the presence of such symptoms as tearing, pain, and inflammation in both eyes. (true or false)

12. Bacterial conjunctivitis is usually treated with:
  a. corticosteroids
  b. topical antibacterial agents
  c. oral antibiotics

13. The two major nursing goals in the care of the child with conjunctivitis are:
  a.

  b.

14. An important nursing consideration in bacterial conjunctivitis is:

15. What are the two types of stomatitis typically seen in children?
  a.

  b.

16. Differentiate between aphthous and herpetic stomatitis by labeling the following clinical manifestations appropriately.
  1. aphthous stomatitis
  2. herpetic stomatitis
  a. ____ a benign but painful condition whose cause is unknown
  b. ____ caused by the herpes simplex virus (HSV)
  c. ____ lesions are small, whitish ulcerations surrounded by red border
  d. ____ commonly called "cold sores" or "fever blisters"
  e. ____ contagious

17. _____ constitute the most common infections in the world.

18. Identify two reasons young children are at risk for parasitic infections.
  a.

  b.

19. Nursing responsibilities related to parasitic intestinal infections are directed toward:
  a.

  b.

  c.

20. The nurse's most important function in relation to parasitic infections is:

21. _____ is the most common intestinal parasitic pathogen in the United States.

22. _____ or _____ is the most common helminthic infection in the United States.

23. ___ The principal symptom of pinworms is intense perianal itching. (true or false)

24. List six symptoms that might indicate the presence of pinworms in a young child who has difficulty verbalizing.
    a.

    b.

    c.

    d.

    e.

    f.

25. The most common test for diagnosing pinworms is the _____.

26. Briefly describe the Poison Prevention Packaging Act of 1970.

27. Identify the developmental characteristics of young children that predispose them to poisoning by ingestion.
    a.

    b.

    c.

    d.

28. List the four principles of emergency treatment following the ingestion of toxic agents.
    a.

    b.

    c.

    d.

29. The preferred method of inducing vomiting at home is through the administration of _____.

30. Identify the indications for gastric lavage.
    a.

    b.

    c.

31. ___ Vomiting is indicated in the treatment of corrosives ingestion. (true or false)

32. The immediate danger from most hydrocarbons is _____.

33. ___ Ingestion of plant parts is one of the most common causes of childhood poisoning. (true or false)

34. ___ Acute salicylate poisoning is considered a more serious intoxication than chronic ingestion. (true or false)

35. _____ is the most common drug poisoning among children and produces _____ damage.

36. Initial management for acetaminophen poisoning is _____ or _____ if the child is treated within 2 hours of the ingestion. If treatment is delayed longer than 2 hours, _____ is administered.

37. When the chronic ingestion of lead stops, it takes the body _____ as long to excrete the stored lead as it did to accumulate it.

38. The most serious and irreversible side effects of lead intoxication are on the _____ system.

39. ___ Erythrocyte protophyrin (EP) level is a sensitive indicator of low lead exposure. (true or false)

40. List four commonly used chelating drugs.
    a.

    b.

    c.

    d.

41. _____ is a broad term that includes intentional physical abuse or neglect, emotional abuse or neglect, and sexual abuse of children, usually by adults.

42. ___ Child neglect involves more children than any other form of child maltreatment. (true or false)

43. What three broad factors seem to predispose children to maltreatment?
    a.

b.

c.

44. The most important criterion on which to base the decision to report child maltreatment is:
    a. inappropriate parental concern for the degree of injury
    b. refusal of parents to sign for additional tests or agree to necessary treatment
    c. incompatibility between the history given and the injury sustained
    d. conflicting stories about the "accident" from parents or child
    e. unavailability of the parents for questioning

45. The physical abuse child victim usually:
    a. belongs to a low socioeconomic population
    b. readily identifies the abusing parent
    c. in no way contributes to the abusing situation
    d. is wary of physical contact with adults

46. Identify three broad nursing goals associated with child maltreatment.
    a.

    b.

    c.

47. List six types of sexual abuse.
    a.

    b.

    c.

    d.

    e.

    f.

IV. Application, Analysis, and Synthesis of Essential Concepts

A. Clinical Situation: Mrs. Braun brings her 4-year-old daughter, Jill, to the pediatric clinic. She tells the nurse practitioner that Jill has been scratching herself around the anus and has been sleeping restlessly. A tentative diagnosis of pinworms infection is made.
    1. How would a diagnosis of pinworms be confirmed.

2. Identify three nursing goals associated with pinworm infection in a child.
    a.

    b.

    c.

B. Experiential Exercise: Spend a day in the Emergency Room to observe the types of poisoning that occur and their emergency treatment. Answer the following questions and include specific examples to illustrate these concepts.
    1. Identify at least three nursing interventions for each of the following areas of emergency treatment.
        a. Assessment–

        b. Gastric decontamination–

        c. Family support–

        d. Prevention of recurrence–

    2. Salicylates and acetaminophen are the two most commonly ingested drugs among children. Match the following statements regarding ingestion with the appropriate drug. Mark A if the answer is acetaminophen and S if the answer is salicylates.
        a. ____ Hyperpnea and hyperpyrexia are common clinical manifestations.
        b. ____ N-acetylcysteine (Mucomyst) is the antidote.
        c. ____ In chronic overdose, it can cause bleeding tendencies.
        d. ____ Bleeding is treated by vitamin K.
        e. ____ Acute overdose results in hepatic damage.

3. What four questions that would assess parents' knowledge should be included in a parent education program regarding accidental poisoning preparedness?

   a.

   b.

   c.

   d.

C. Experiential Exercise: Assess a specific child's environment with regard to its potential for lead poisoning. Answer the following questions and include specific examples that illustrate these concepts.

1. When assessing the child's environment, what environmental factors would alert the nurse to the potential for lead poisoning?

   a.

   b.

   c.

   d.

   e.

2. What early signs of lead poisoning should the nurse be alert to when performing an assessment?

   a. Behavioral changes–

   b. Other manifestations–

3. If, during the assessment, the presence of lead poisoning is suspected, what should the nurse's initial goal be?

4. Blood lead level determines the degree of risk and the type of intervention for the child with lead poisoning. At what level does the child require each of the following?

   a. environmental evaluation and remediation _____

   b. chelation therapy _____
   c. emergency intervention _____

5. The three modes of therapy for a child with lead poisoning are:

   a.

   b.

   c.

6. Since lead poisoning can occur in children from all socioeconomic strata, what factors regarding food preparation and diet would you include in a preventive teaching plan for parents of young children?

   a.

   b.

   c.

   d.

   e.

D. Experiential Exercise: Care for a child who is hospitalized as a result of maltreatment. Answer the following questions and include specific examples that illustrate these concepts.

1. Identify characteristics in each of the following areas that can be used to assess the vulnerability of families to abuse.

   a. Parents–

   b. Child–

   c. Environment–

2. What two factors are used as diagnostic tools in determining child abuse?

   a.

   b.

3. Identify at least five areas that should arouse suspicion of abuse when the nurse is obtaining a history.

   a.

   b.

   c.

   d.

   e.

4. Develop three nursing diagnoses that could be used as a basis for the care of an abusing family.

   a.

   b.

   c.

5. Why are accurate nurses' notes essential to any suspected maltreatment situation?

6. For each of the following nursing goals, identify one evaluation criterion that indicates that achievement of these goals.

   a. Protect from further abuse—

   b. Prevent recurrence—

   c. Relieve or reduce anxiety and stress—

   d. Prevent abuse—

   e. Support parents—

   f. Educate parents regarding normal child growth and development—

V. Suggested Readings

Hussey GD, Klein M: A randomized, controlled trial of vitamin A in children with severe measles, N Engl J Med 323(3):160-164, 1990.

> Since measles kills about 2 million children annually, this research study revealed significant findings. The conclusion of the study is that treatment with vitamin A reduces morbidity and mortality of children with severe measles.

Jones SH, Jenista JA: Fifth disease: role for nurses in pediatric practice, Pediatr Nurs 16(2):148-149, 1990.

> The authors discuss the common childhood disease caused by the parvovirus B19 (fifth disease). Though mild in children, the disease is a danger to pregnant women. Nurses must recognize and intervene to protect high-risk individuals.

Kurt TL: The (internal) dangers of acrylic fingernails, JAMA 263(16):2181, 1990, (letter).

> This letter to the editor raises a significant issue regarding the danger to children of solutions used in the application and removal of acrylic fingernails. Ingestion of these solvents must be treated differently from that of conventional nail polish removers. Safety issues regarding protection of children are obvious.

Lewis L: Establishing a therapeutic relationship with an abused child, Pediatr Nurs 16(3):263-264, 1990.

> The author gives specific guidelines for nurses to establish a therapeutic relationship with a child who has been abused. A step-by-step process that includes language, setting, and developmentally compatible approaches and interventions is presented. An excellent article for any pediatric nurse who may care for abused children.

Shannon MW, Graef JW: Lead intoxication in infancy, Pediatrics 89(1):87-90, 1992.

> This study of 50 new infants (median age of 11 months) in a Massachusetts lead referral program concluded that lead intoxication in infants is common and has significantly different origins from that in toddlers. Lead intoxication in infant formula reconstituted with contaminated water may account for many of the cases. It is thus recommended that lead screening begin at the age of 6 months for children with any likelihood of lead exposure.

Chapter 15

Health Promotion of the School–Age Child and Family

I. Chapter Overview

Chapter 15 discusses the school-age period, the ages from 6 to 12. Because this developmental stage is characterized by greater social awareness and social skills, it is important for nursing students to understand the roles of peer and family relationships, school, and play in the socialization process. At the completion of this chapter, the student will have a knowledge of the child's growth and development and be aware of areas of special concern to parents. This knowledge will enable the student to develop nursing goals and interventions that foster health maintenance behavior in school-age children and their families.

II. Learning Objectives

Upon completion of this chapter, it is expected that the student will be able to:

1. Describe the physical, cognitive, and moral changes that take place during the middle childhood years.

2. Describe ways to help a child develop a sense of accomplishment.

3. Demonstrate an understanding of the changing interpersonal relationships of school-age children.

4. Discuss the role of the peer group in the socialization of the school-age child.

5. Discuss the role of schools in the development and socialization of the school-age child.

6. Outline an appropriate health teaching plan for the school-age child.

7. Plan a sex education session for a group of school-age children.

8. Identify the causes and discuss the preventive aspects of injury in middle childhood.

III. Review of Essential Concepts

1. With _____ children of this age establish the first close relationships outside the family group.

2. The middle years begin with the shedding of the _____ and end at puberty with the acquisition of the final _____.

3. ___ During the school-age years, a child will grow approximately 2 inches per year and will almost triple in weight. (true or false)

4. Identify the three most pronounced physiologic changes that indicate increasing maturity in the school-age child.

   a.

   b.

   c.

5. The average age of puberty in girls is _____, and in boys it is _____.
6. According to Freud, the school-age child is in the _____ stage.
   a. oral
   b. anal
   c. oedipal
   d. latency
7. According to Erikson, the developmental task of middle childhood is acquiring a sense of:
   a. trust
   b. autonomy
   c. initiative
   d. industry
8. Failure to develop a sense of accomplishment results in a sense of _____.
9. ___ In the process of self-evaluation, children actively strive to reach internalized goals or levels of attainment that they hope to achieve. (true or false)
10. According to Piaget, the school-age child is in the _____ stage.
    a. sensorimotor
    b. preoperational
    c. concrete operational
    d. formal operational
11. ___ During this cognitive stage, children progress from making judgments based on what they see (perceptual) to making judgments based on what they reason (conceptual). (true or false)
12. One of the major cognitive tasks of school-age children is mastering the concepts of _____.
13. Define the term classification.

14. ___ The most significant skill acquired during the school-age years is the ability to read. (true or false)
15. _____ is the statement that best describes the younger school-age child's perception of rules and judgment of actions.
    a. Judges an act by its intentions rather than by the consequences alone
    b. Believes that rules and judgments are not absolute
    c. Understands the reason behind rules
    d. Interprets accidents and misfortunes as punishment for misdeeds
16. _____ best describes the older school-age child's perception of rules and judgment of actions.
    a. Does not understand the reasons for rules
    b. Takes into account different points of view to make a judgment
    c. Judges an act by its consequences
    d. Believes that rules and judgments are absolute
17. Identification with _____ appears to be a strong influence in the child's attainment of independence from parents.
18. ___ During the early school years, children display considerable differences relative to gender in their play experiences. (true or false)
19. Identify three valuable lessons that children learn from daily interactions with age-mates.
    a.

    b.

    c.

20. One of the outstanding characteristics of middle childhood is the formation of _____ or _____.
21. A complex form of group play that evolves from group games is _____ or _____.
22. Identify the three significant characteristics of team membership that are relevant to child development.
    a.

    b.

    c.

23. Define self-concept:

24. Until the child enters school, the primary sphere of influence is the _____.
25. _____ serve as models with whom children identify and whom they try to emulate.
26. List four specific guidelines that parents can use to help their children in school.
    a.

    b.

    c.

    d.

27. Identify the signs of stress children may exhibit.

28. What two factors are contributing to an increase in childhood obesity?
    a.

    b.

29. Match the following behavior with the ages at which they are exhibited.
    a. ___ centers life around school
    b. ___ enjoys group activities involving both sexes
    c. ___ enjoys sports
    d. ___ loves friends; talks incessantly about them
       a. 6 years
       b. 9 years
       c. 12 years

30. ___ The appearance of permanent teeth in the school-age child begins with the eruption of the 6-year-molar. (true or false)

31. Before providing information on sexuality to parents and children, the nurse must first be knowledgeable about:
    a.

    b.

    c.

32. ___ The most common cause of severe accidental injury and death in school-age children is motor vehicle accidents. (true or false)

IV. Application, Analysis, and Synthesis of Essential Concepts

A. Clinical Situation: Jimmy Douglas, age 9, is brought to the pediatrician's office by his mother for his annual physical examination. His height and weight are obtained. Jimmy's height is 52 in. (132.2 cm) and his weight is 62 lb (28.13 kg). Jimmy's vision is evaluated as 20/30 in both eyes.
    1. Plot Jimmy's height and weight on a growth chart. How do his measurements compare with the norms for this age?

a. Height–

b. Weight–

2. Mrs. Douglas tells the nurse that Jimmy likes to help his father with the yard work. However, Jimmy's work is not always up to his father's expectations. What advice could be given?

3. Mrs. Douglas expresses concern because she is having a problem with dishonesty in her 6-year-old daughter. What information could the nurse provide to assist Mrs. Douglas in dealing with this concern?

4. Mrs. Douglas asks the nurse for suggestions that will foster Jimmy's development. What should the nurse's response be?
    a.

    b.

    c.

    d.

    e.

    f.

B. Experiential Exercise: Interview a school-age child and his parents about changing interpersonal relationships and peer groups. Answer the following questions and include specific responses to illustrate the concepts.
    1. Why do school-age children spend an increased amount of time away from their homes and families?

2. Why are relationships with age-mates an important social interaction in the life of the school-age child?

3. What is the function of gang membership for the school-age child?

V. Suggested Readings

American Academy of Pediatrics, Committee on Accident and Poison Prevention: Bicycle helmets, Pediatrics 85:229-230, 1990.

> The committee on Accident and Poison Prevention includes five recommendations for the use of bicycle helmets in children. The committee highly recommends this practice to prevent injury.

Konguth ML: School illnesses: who's absent and why? Pediatr Nurs 16(1):95-99: 1990.

> This study explores the excessive absences of children from school. Absent children were predominantly female, of minority status, and poor. Absence from school results in educational and social inequity. School nurses can effectively intervene to alter the frequency and length of absentism in this population.

Vessey, JA, and others: Teaching children about their internal bodies, Pediatr Nurs 16(1):29-33, 1990.

> These authors discuss appropriate and effective methods, language, and timing for nurses to teach basic anatomy and physiology to early school-age children.

Wall-Haas CL: Nurses' attitudes toward sexuality in adolescent patients, Pediatr Nurs 17(6):549-555, 1991.

> This descriptive study is a survey of the sexual attitudes and nursing practice of 39 nurses who care for adolescents in a large metropolitan teaching hospital. The results reveal that, although the nurses recognized the importance of sexuality for the adolescent patient and were theoretically capable of addressing issues of adolescent sexuality, they were uncomfortable incorporating issues of sexuality, counseling, and education into their nursing practice.

Chapter 16
Health Promotion of the Adolescent and Family

I. Chapter Overview

Chapter 16 examines the frequently perplexing adolescent period. Since this is often a time of difficult transition from childhood to adulthood, students need to be aware of problematic behavior that may occur. At the completion of this chapter, the student will understand the interplay of physical, psychosocial, and emotional factors in the adolescent's development and interpersonal relations. This knowledge will enable the student to provide anticipatory guidance to assist the child and family with the intricate developmental issues of adolescence.

II. Learning Objectives

Upon completion of this chapter, it is expected that the reader will be able to:

1. Describe the physical changes that occur at puberty in the male and female.

2. Discuss the reactions of the adolescent to physical changes that take place at puberty.

3. Demonstrate an understanding of the processes by which the adolescent develops a sense of identity.

4. Discuss the significance of the changing interpersonal relationships and the role of the peer group during adolescence.

5. Outline a health teaching plan for adolescents.

6. Plan a sex education session for a group of adolescents.

7. Identify the causes and discuss the preventive aspects of injuries during adolescence.

III. Review of Essential Concepts

1. Adolescence is customarily viewed as beginning with the gradual appearance of _____ and ending with cessation of _____.
2. Differentiate between the following terms:
    a. Puberty—

    b. Adolescence—

3. The physical changes of puberty are primarily the result of _____ _____ influenced by the central nervous system.
4. Identify the two most obvious physical changes that occur during adolescence.
    a.

    b.

5. Differentiate between the following two terms.

   a. Primary sex characteristics—

   b. Secondary sex characteristics—

6. _____ and _____ are the two types of sex hormones that are responsible for the variety of biologic changes observed during pubescence and puberty.

7. Most of the physical growth of adolescents occurs during a 24- to 36-month period known as the adolescent _____.

8. The normal age range of menarche is usually considered to be _____ to _____ years; the average age is _____ years.

9. The overt sign that indicates puberty in boys is the beginning of _____ of seminal fluid.

10. Skeletal growth differences between boys and girls are reflected in greater overall _____ and longer _____ in boys. There is also an increase in _____ width in boys and greater _____ in girls.

11. ___ Enlargement of the larynx and vocal cords occurs in both boys and girls to produce voice changes. (true or false)

12. _____ glands become extremely active during puberty, contributing to the pathogenesis of _____.

13. ___ Adult values for the formed elements of the blood, respiratory rate, and basal metabolic rate are attained during adolescence. (true or false)

14. According to Erikson, the developmental crisis of adolescence is developing a sense of:
    a. industry
    b. identity
    c. initiative
    d. autonomy

15. A sense of _____ identity appears to be an essential precursor of the sense of _____ identity.

16. The group offers an identity to the young adolescent in terms of _____.

17. When does role diffusion occur?

18. Adolescents encounter expectations for mature sex-role behavior from both _____ and _____.

19. Adolescents are unstable emotionally. They vacillate quickly between _____ behavior and _____ behavior.

20. According to Piaget, the adolescent is in the stage of _____.

21. Identify five characteristics that are typical of the adolescent's thought processes.
    a.

    b.

    c.

    d.

    e.

22. The _____ has an intense influence on an adolescent's self-evaluation and behavior.

23. Statistics reveal that _____ of all teens have had sex by age 17.

24. Nurses need to recognize _____ attraction and to be sensitive to the fact that not all youths are involved in heterosexual relationships.

25. ___ It has been determined that the body image established during adolescence is temporary and subject to change. (true or false)

26. At the end of the adolescent period, the child should be able to:
    a.

    b.

    c.

    d.

    e.

    f.

27. ___ The increase in height, weight, muscle mass, and sexual maturity of adolescence is accompanied by greater nutritional requirements. (true or false)

28. List the mineral deficiencies that are most likely to characterize the adolescent diet.
    a.

    b.

    c.

29. Adolescent involvement in sports contributes to:

a.

b.

c.

30. What type of visual disturbance is most common during adolescence?

31. List five major areas of stress for the adolescent.

a.

b.

c.

d.

e.

32. Sex education programs should present content from six aspects:

a.

b.

c.

d.

e.

f.

33. The greatest single cause of death in the adolescent age group is_____.

34. Almost half of the fatalities in the adolescent age group are related to _____.

35. What three factors contribute to the problem of motor vehicle injuries in adolescence?

a.

b.

c.

IV. Application, Analysis, and Synthesis of Essential Concepts

A. Clinical Situation: Alice Spears is a 14-year-old who comes to the pediatric clinic for a yearly checkup. She is accompanied by her mother. Although she has felt well recently, Alice is concerned because she is overweight and has recently developed acne. She also began menstruating 6 months ago.

1. Alice's height is 64 in. (162.7 cm) and her weight is 161 lb (73.08 kg). How do her measurements compare with those of other girls her age?

a. Height—

b. Weight—

2. What principles of physical growth should be explained to Alice since she is concerned about her weight?

B. Experiential Exercise: Interview the parents of an adolescent about the teenager's involvement in peer groups, relationship with parents, and sense of identity. Answer the following questions and include specific responses that illustrate these concepts.

1. How does the peer group contribute to the development of a sense of identity in the adolescent?

2. Identify some ways in which group identity is demonstrated by the adolescent.

a.

b.

c.

d.

3. Why are peer groups an important influence during the adolescent years?

4. What six factors would the nurse offer to the parents to enable them to better relate to their adolescent?

   a.

   b.

   c.

   d.

   e.

   f.

C. Experiential Exercise: Interview an adolescent about his health promotion behavior. Answer the following questions and include specific responses to illustrate these concepts.

1. Why is adequate intake of the following minerals necessary during adolescence?

   a. Calcium–

   b. Iron–

   c. Zinc–

2. Why is fatigue a common complaint of adolescence?

3. What can be gained from participation in sports?

   a.

   b.

   c.

4. Why should the nurse promote dental hygiene in the adolescent?

5. What are the most common types of accidents that occur during the adolescent years?

   a.

   b.

   c.

   d.

   e.

   f.

6. What developmental characteristics predispose the adolescent to accidents?

7. What elements should the nurse include in a sex education program for adolescents?

   a.

   b.

   c.

   d.

   e.

8. For each of the following nursing goals, develop nursing interventions that will promote optimal health in the adolescent.

   a. Promote adequate nutritional intake—

   b. Promote the development of proper sleep habits—

   c. Promote optimal physical activity—

   d. Promote good personal hygiene practices—

   e. Prevent physical injury—

V. Suggested Readings

American Academy of Pediatrics, Committee on Communications: Impact of rock lyrics and music videos on children and youth, Pediatrics 83(2):314-315, 1989.

> The Committee on Communications explores the issues of rock music and music videos and includes a set of recommendations regarding each issue.

Blum RW: Global trends in adolescent health, JAMA 265(20):2711-2719, 1991.

> This article contains reviews of the morbidity and mortality trends for adolescents throughout the world. The authors discuss demographic trends, educational trends, major causes of morbidity, major causes of mortality, and health concerns of youths from their own perspective. An interesting and comprehensive discussion.

Sheehan, MK, Ostwald SK, Rothenberger J: Perceptions of sexual responsibility: do young men and women agree? Pediatr Nurs 12:17-21, 1986.

> These authors investigated the perception of responsibility for contraception among late adolescents to determine whether age, gender, or sexual activity influences perceptions of responsibility and to explore the relationship between this perceived responsibility and subsequent contraceptive choice. The authors found that older adolescents perceived contraception as a shared responsibility but that they were unlikely to use contraception during their first intercourse. The implications of the findings for sex education are discussed.

Chapter 17
Health Problems of Middle Childhood and Adolescence

I. Chapter Overview

Chapter 17 introduces nursing considerations that are integral to the care of the middle child and the adolescent experiencing physical health problems. Although this age group is usually healthy, students need to be aware of the common health problems related to the physical changes and other potentially serious illnesses or injuries that may affect them. At the completion of this chapter, the student will understand the commonly encountered physical health deviations of the middle child and the adolescent and recognize the potential for secondary psychologic problems. This knowledge will provide a basis for the student to develop nursing goals and interventions to support and educate the middle child, the adolescent, and the family.

II. Learning Objectives

Upon completion of this chapter, it is expected that the student will be able to:

1. Outline a plan of care for the child or adolescent with a health problem.

2. Describe the most common causes of growth and/or maturation failure in later childhood.

3. Demonstrate an understanding of common disorders of the male and female reproductive systems.

4. Demonstrate an understanding of health problems related to sexuality.

5. Outline a plan of care for the child or adolescent with an eating disorder.

6. Discuss the manifestations and nursing management of selected emotional and/or behavioral problems.

III. Review of Essential Concepts

1. The principal cause of infectious mononucleosis is the _____ virus.

2. The early symptoms of mononucleosis are:
   a.

   b.

   c.

   d.

   e.

   f.

   g.

3. The _____, a slide test of high specificity, is used in the diagnosis of infectious mononucleosis.

4. What factors are related to the onset of smoking during adolescence?

5. List the four stages of the process of becoming a smoker.
   a.

   b.

   c.

   d.

6. ___ The use of smokeless tobacco products is a safe substitute for cigarette smoking. (true or false)

7. Two recent areas of focus for smoking prevention programs are:
   a.

   b.

8. The role of health professionals in relation to sports injuries is directed toward _____, _____, _____, and _____. Of these, which is the most important?

9. Identify three examples of overuse injuries.
   a.

   b.

   c.

10. Stress fractures occur as a result of:

11. Management of overuse syndromes is directed toward:
   a.

   b.

   c.

12. ___ Prevention of sports injuries is probably the most important aspect of any athletic program. (true or false)

13. The most common cause of short stature and/or developmental delay is _____ _____.

14. Identify the three outstanding features of girls with Turner syndrome.
   a.

   b.

   c.

15. Characteristic features of boys with Klinefelter syndrome include:
   a.

   b.

   c.

   d.

   e.

16. ___ The most common cause of secondary amenorrhea during adolescence is inhibition of the secretion of pituitary hormones. (true or false)

17. The treatment of choice for dysmenorrhea in adolescents is the administration of drugs that block the formation of _____.

18. The most frequent problems related to the reproductive organs of the male in later childhood are:
   a.

   b.

   c.

   d.

   e.

19. The most important nursing goal in nursing care of the pregnant teenager is:

20. For a contraceptive method to be safe and effective, it must be _____.

21. List the methods of contraception available to the adolescent.
   a.

   b.

   c.

   d.

e.

f.

g.

22. The most prevalent sexually transmitted diseases in the adolescent and adult population are _____ and _____ infections.

23. The two sexually transmitted diseases that do not have a cure are:
a.

b.

24. Match the following sexually transmitted diseases with their causative organisms and the drug of choice for treatment. (Answers may be used more than once.)
a. ___ gonorrhea
b. ___ chlamydial infection
c. ___ herpes pro genitalis
d. ___syphilis
e. ___moniliasis
f. ___ trichomoniasis
  1) *C. trachomatis*
  2) herpesvirus hominis type II
  3) *Trichomonas vaginalis*
  4) *Neisseria gonorrhoeae*
  5) *Treponema pallidum*
  6) *Candida albicans*
  7) metronidazole
  8) tetracycline
  9) acyclovir
  10) nystatin
  11) penicillin

25. The complication of pelvic inflammatory disease that is of major concern is:

26. ____ More than half of rape victims are between 15 and 19 years of age. (true or false)

27. During the initial contact with the adolescent rape victim, it is important that she know she is:
a.

b.

28. The two phases of the rape trauma syndrome are:
a.

b.

29. _____ is an increase in body weight resulting from an excessive accumulation of fat or, simply, the state of being too fat.

30. _____ is the state of weighing more than average for height and body build, which may or may not include an increased amount of fat.

31. What is the cause of obesity?

32. Recent theories that tend to explain the development of obesity are:
a.

b.

33. ___ As a rule, children who are 10% over normal for their height and weight should be further evaluated. (true or false)

34. The goals of a weight-loss program include:
a.

b.

c.

d.

35. In the management of obesity, it has been observed that:
a. Weight loss will occur only when caloric expenditure is greater than caloric intake.
b. There is little correlation between motivation to lose weight and the success of the weight-reduction program.
c. The most successful diets are those which require the avoidance of specific foods.
d. The alteration of eating behavior has little effect in maintaining long-term weight control.

36. _____ is a disorder characterized by severe weight loss in the absence of obvious physical cause, in which emaciation occurs as a result of self-inflicted starvation.

37. The onset of anorexia nervosa generally takes place at or near _____.

38. Identify the characteristics frequently displayed by young women with anorexia nervosa.
a.

b.

c.

d.

39. The two dominant psychologic aspects of anorexia nervosa are:

a.

b.

40. List the clinical manifestations of anorexia nervosa.

a.

b.

c.

d.

e.

f.

g.

h.

i.

41. _____ is an eating disorder characterized by binge eating and purging.

42. Purging methods employed by bulimics include _____, _____, _____ and rigorous exercise.

43. Briefly describe the two categories of bulimics.

a.

b.

44. ___ Medical complications occur in bulimics primarily as a result of their frequent vomiting. (true or false)

45. Identify two nursing interventions that are important during the acute phase of treatment of bulimia.

a.

b.

46. Define attention deficit hyperactivity disorder.

47. List the components of the multiple approach to the management of attention deficit disorder.

a.

b.

c.

d.

48. Define enuresis:

49. List the various therapeutic techniques that can be employed to manage enuresis.

a.

b.

c.

d.

e.

50. Define encopresis:

51. _____ is the more descriptive term now used for encopresis when psychiatric dysfunction does not contribute to the soiling.

52. Predisposing factors for encopresis seem to be:_____ and _____.

53. What are the three stages of response in posttraumatic stress disorder?

a.

b.

c.

54. What is the primary nursing goal in the management of school phobia?

55. Recurrent abdominal pain is almost always attributed to a _____ etiology.

56. ___ Depression in the child is easy to detect. (true or false)

57. List behavioral characteristics of children with depression.
    a.

    b.

    c.

    d.

    e.

    f.

    g.

58. Childhood schizophrenia is a term used to describe _____ in ego functioning that appear after the first 4 to 5 years of life.

59. _____ and _____ are the drugs most often abused by adolescents.

60. _____ is the most powerful antifatigue agent.

61. A major factor in the treatment and rehabilitation of the young drug user is careful _____ to determine the _____ the drug plays in the youngster's life.

62. ____ Suicide is the third leading cause of death during the adolescent years. (true or false)

63. Distinguish between the following terms:
    a. Suicide gesture–

    b. Suicide attempt–

64. _____ is the method of choice for most adolescents who attempt suicide.

65. ___ Most adolescents' suicidal gestures are impulsive acts committed to force parents or other significant persons to pay attention to their need for help. (true or false)

66. Nursing care of the suicidal adolescent includes:
    a.

    b.

    c.

IV. Application, Analysis, and Synthesis of Essential Concepts

A. Clinical Situation: Rosemary, age 16, is admitted to the adolescent unit with a severe sore throat, persistent fever, fatigue, and general malaise. A diagnosis of infectious mononucleosis is made.
1. How was the diagnosis of infectious mononucleosis established?

2. What might the nurse tell Rosemary about the usual course of infectious mononucleosis in the following areas?
   a. Acute symptoms–

   b. Persistent fatigue–

   c. Restricted activity–

3. What therapeutic measures may be used to relieve Rosemary's sore throat?

4. What are the nursing goals in caring for Rosemary?
   a.

   b.

B. Clinical Situation: Derek, age 15, has been experiencing a deep, persistent, dull ache over the left tibia that progressed to pain with each heel strike during a cross-country meet. The coach refers Derek to the sports medicine team at University Medical Center for evaluation. A stress fracture of the left tibia is discovered.
1. What two general types of injury are related to sports?
   a.

   b.

2. Rest is the primary therapy for overuse syndromes. How is this treatment modality likely to be interpreted in Derek's case?

3. What is the major goal of the therapeutic management of overuse syndromes such as Derek's stress fracture?

4. Derek asks the nurse on the sports medicine team if she thinks running is a good sport for him. What should the nurse assess to answer this question?

5. What nursing interventions might the nurse on the sports medicine team employ to prevent sports injuries?
   a.

   b.

   c.

   d.

C. Experiential Exercise: Spend a day in a gynecology clinic to oversee the management of sexually transmitted diseases and other disorders affecting the female reproductive system. Answer the following questions and include specific examples to illustrate these concepts.
   1. What two problems in the female adolescent most frequently require attention from health professionals?
      a.

      b.

   2. What are four advantages of undergoing the initial pelvic examination in early adolescence?
      a.

      b.

      c.

      d.

   3. Define the following terms to differentiate their meanings:

   a. Primary amenorrhea—

   b. Secondary amenorrhea—

   4. Identify the most common causes of secondary dysmenorrhea in adolescents.
      a.

      b.

D. Experiential Exercise: Role-play an interaction between a nurse and an anorexic or bulimic adolescent to demonstrate the adolescent's perception of her disorder and how the nurse would counsel her.
   1. What usually precedes the onset of anorexia nervosa?

   2. What contemporary trends are considered factors in the greatly increased incidence of anorexia and bulimia?
      a.

      b.

   3. The following are characteristics associated with anorexia nervosa and/or bulimia. Mark A if the item is related to anorexia, B if it applies to bulimia, and A,B if it may be associated with both disorders.
      a. ___ binge-eating
      b. ___ self-induced vomiting
      c. ___ self-imposed starvation
      d. ___ awareness of abnormality of eating pattern
      e. ___ denial of existence of hunger
      f. ___ cold intolerance
      g. ___ normal or slightly above normal weight
      h. ___ emaciated appearance
      i. ___ increased incidence of dental caries
      j. ___ distinctive hand lesions
      k. ___ control as a major issue
      l. ___ secondary amenorrhea
   4. Behavior modification may be employed in the treatment of both anorexia nervosa and

bulimia. Identify the essential aspects of such a program.

a.

b.

c.

d.

e.

E. Experiential Exercise: Interview an obese adolescent to assess eating patterns. Answer the following questions and include specific responses that illustrate these concepts.
1. Why is obesity considered a major problem of adolescence?

2. Identify six factors that may contribute to the development of obesity.
a.

b.

c.

d.

e.

f.

3. Identify six behaviors that are characteristic of the eating pattern of obese adolescents.
a.

b.

c.

d.

e.

f.

4. Formulate five nursing diagnoses that could apply to the obese adolescent.
a.

b.

c.

d.

e.

F. Clinical Situation: Michelle is a 16-year-old girl who is admitted to the adolescent unit following the ingestion of 10 of her mother's barbiturates with an unknown quantity of alcohol. Michelle is known to be a "problem drinker." When she recovers consciousness after gastric lavage, Michelle sobs that she wishes she were dead because she has broken up with her boyfriend.
1. In what category might this suicide attempt be classified?

2. In what ways was Michelle's suicide attempt a typical one for an adolescent girl?

3. In assessing Michelle's family status, what factors is the nurse likely to discover?

V. Suggested Readings

American Academy of Pediatrics, Committee on Adolescence: Contraception and adolescents, Pediatrics 86(1):134-138, 1990.

> The Committee on Adolescence discusses parameters regarding adolescent sexual behavior: adolescent sexual behavior, adolescent contraceptive behavior, role of the pediatrician, counseling of adolescents about contraception, and methods of contraception. A set of five recommendations concludes the discussion.

Clubb RL: Promoting non-tobacco use in childhood, Pediatr Nurs 17(6):566-570, 1991.

> The author discusses both the availability of cigarettes and smokeless tobacco to children and some hypotheses regarding why children start to smoke. The author explores the value of smoking prevention programs designed

around the framework of social learning theory. The nurse's strategic position to plan, deliver, and evaluate smoking prevention programs is emphasized.

Epstein LH, and others: Ten-year follow-up behavioral family-based treatment for obese children, JAMA 264(19):2519-2523, 1990.

This article is a report on a study done on 76 obese children and their parents over a 10-year period. A family-based behavioral therapy was used to alter the weight gain in both child and parents. Results of this study provide, according to the authors, the first evidence for long-term treatment of childhood obesity from preadolescence through young adulthood. Nurses will be interested in one of the conclusions of this study: behavioral treatments that focus on changing eating, exercise, and behavioral skills are related to long-term success in treating obese children.

Sherts-Engel NC: Levonorgestrel subdermal implants (Norplant) for long-term contraception, MCN 16:232, 1991.

A very brief presentation of Norplant and its use as a contraceptive.

Smitherman CH: A drug to ease attention deficit-disorder, MCN 15(6):363-365, 1990.

A contemporary and thorough exploration of attention deficit-hyperactivity disorder (ADHD). All aspects of the use of methylphenidate hydrochloride (Ritalin) to treat children with this disorder are presented. The content in this article is a must for any nurse working with children with this disorder. Guidelines for family assessment is an especially useful addition to this article.

Chapter 18
Impact of Chronic Illness, Disability, or Death on the Child and Family

I. Chapter Overview

Chapter 18 introduces nursing considerations essential to the care of the child with a chronic illness or disability. Since nursing students will be required to care for children with special needs, it is important that they understand the family's reaction to the loss of a "perfect" child and become familiar with the process of adjusting to a disability. At the completion of this chapter, the student should understand the impact that a diagnosis of a chronic illness or disability has on both the child and family and be able to develop appropriate nursing interventions to assist each family member to adjust and develop to his fullest potential despite the disability.

II. Learning Objectives

Upon completion of this chapter, it is expected that the student will be able to:

1. Identify the scope of and changing trends in care of children with special needs.

2. Define the stages of adjustment to the diagnosis of a chronic condition.

3. Define the stages of grief for the anticipated or actual loss of a child.

4. Identify the major reactions of and effects on the family with a child with a special need.

5. Recognize the impact of the illness or disability on the developmental stages of childhood.

6. Outline nursing interventions that promote the family's optimum adjustment to the child's chronic disorder.

7. Outline nursing interventions that support the family at the time of death.

III. Review of Essential Concepts

1. Match each of the following terms with the appropriate definition.
   a. ___ chronic illness
   b. ___ disability
   c. ___ developmental disability
   d. ___ handicap
      1) broadly refers to a loss of function
      2) refers to environmental barriers that prevent or make difficult full participation or integration
      3) a condition that interferes with daily functioning for more than 3 months in a year, causes hospitalization of more than 1 month in a year, or is likely to do either of these
      4) any severe, chronic disability attributable to a mental or physical impairment or a combination of both that is manifested before age 22 years, is likely to continue indefinitely, and will result in substantial limitation of function

2. ___ Two thirds of all cases of chronic illness are attributable to asthma and congenital heart defects. (true or false)

3. Identify and explain the changing trends in the care of children with special needs.

   a.

   b.

   c.

4. _____ refers to the integration of children with special needs into regular classrooms.

5. The family of the child with special needs is faced with the crisis of:

   a.

   b.

6. List the sequence of stages through which a family progresses following the diagnosis of a chronic illness or disability.

   a.

   b.

   c.

   d.

7. The two most common responses manifested during the adjustment stage are:

   a.

   b.

8. Describe the four types of parental reactions to the child that may occur during the period of adjustment.

   a. Overprotection–

   b. Rejection–

   c. Denial–

   d. Gradual acceptance–

9. Explain the concept of "chronic sorrow."

10. What is the best predictor of long-term marital adjustment of the parents of a child with special needs?

11. ___ Fathers and mothers of a child with special needs adjust and cope differently. (true or false)

12. The most important factors in sibling adjustment to a child with special needs appear to be parental _____, _____, and _____.

13. List three variables that influence the resolution of a crisis following the diagnosis of a serious health problem.

   a.

   b.

   c.

14. Identify the five stages that the family and the terminally ill child experience during anticipatory grief.

   a.

   b.

   c.

   d.

   e.

15. Identify the stages of mourning.

   a.

   b.

   c.

   d.

16. Identify four variables which influence a child's reaction to chronic illness or disability.

a.

b.

c.

d.

17. ___ The impact of a chronic illness or disability is influenced by the age of onset. (true or false)

18. Identify the coping patterns used by children with special needs.
   a.

   b.

   c.

   d.

   e.

19. ___ The concept of death parallels cognitive and psychosocial development. (true or false)

20. The abstract adult meaning of death as irreversible, inevitable, and universal is not understood by most children until _____.

21. For the preschool child, the greatest fear concerning death is _____.

22. Nursing care varies according to the particular disability appearing at the time of birth. Identify six situations that would require special nursing intervention to support the family.
   a.

   b.

   c.

   d.

   e.

   f.

23. List the three most common responses of families to the diagnosis of a disability.
   a.

   b.

   c.

24. List the principles of normalization.
   a.

   b.

   c.

   d.

   e.

25. To foster a realistic adjustment of the family with a special needs child, the nurse must educate the family. This education should include:
   a.

   b.

   c.

26. Identify at least three support strategies the nurse can use to avoid burnout when caring for terminally ill children and their families.
   a.

   b.

   c.

   d.

   e.

   f.

IV. Application, Analysis, and Synthesis of Essential Concepts

A. Experiential Exercise: Spend a morning at a clinic or school for children with disabilities to observe various treatment modalities and programs. Answer the following questions and include specific examples to illustrate these concepts.

1. Describe the four major changes that have occurred in the provision of services to children with special needs.
   a.

   b.

c.

d.

2. How have the above changes served to improve the care of children with special needs?

a.

b.

c.

d.

B. Experiential Exercise: Care for a child who has recently been diagnosed as having a chronic illness or disability.

1. Why is it important for the nurse to understand the responses of family members to a diagnosis of a chronic illness or disability?

a.

b.

c.

2. Briefly describe the stages through which a family progresses following the diagnosis of a chronic illness or disability.
a. Shock and denial–

b. Adjustment–

c. Reintegration and acknowledgment–

d. Freezing-out phase–

3. List nine examples of behavior that should alert the nurse to the presence of denial.

a.

b.

c.

d.

e.

f.

g.

h.

i.

4. Why is it important for the nurse to allow denial to occur for a reasonable period?

a.

b.

5. Briefly describe the reactions and effects of a diagnosis of chronic illness or disability on the following family members:

a. Parents—

b. Siblings—

C. Experiential Exercise: Interview the parents of a child with a disability to determine the family's adjustment. Answer the following questions and include specific responses to illustrate these concepts.

1. Identify the areas the nurse should assess when determining the adequacy of a family's support systems.

   a.

   b.

   c.

2. Why is it necessary for the nurse to assess the family's specific perceptions concerning the illness or disability?

3. Briefly describe some of the behaviors that might be observed in a child who has adjusted well to his disability.

   a.

   b.

   c.

4. What are the basic nursing goals for families and children with special needs?

   a.

   b.

   c.

   d.

   e.

5. What areas must the nurse assess before developing a plan of care for a disabled child and her family?

   a.

   b.

   c.

   d.

   e.

   f.

6. For each of the following nursing goals, identify at least three appropriate nursing interventions that can be used to promote reality adjustment.

   a. Supply information—

   b. Promote normal development—

   c. Establish realistic future goals—

D. Experiential Exercise: Interview children in various age groups to determine their perceptions of death. Answer the following questions and include specific responses to illustrate these concepts.

1. How do children between the ages of 3 and 5 years of age view death?

   a.

   b.

   c.

2. If a preschooler becomes seriously ill, how is he likely to perceive the illness?

3. By _____ or _____ years of age, most children have an adult concept of death.

4. Why do adolescents have the most difficulty in coping with death, especially their own?

5. Identify at least eight nursing interventions that could be used when caring for a terminally ill adolescent in the hospital.

a.

b.

c.

d.

e.

f.

g.

h.

E. Experiential Exercise: Care for a child who is hospitalized with a life-threatening illness.

  1. Briefly describe the following five stages through which a family proceeds when there is anticipated loss of a child.

    a. Denial–

    b. Anger–

    c. Bargaining–

  d. Depression–

  e. Acceptance–

2. How does the grief process in the surviving family members differ when the child's death is unexpected as opposed to expected?

F. Experiential Exercise: Care for a child with a chronic illness and his family.

  1. List the nursing goals that are appropriate to the nursing diagnosis "Self-care deficit related to specific impairment."

    a.

    b.

  2. What interventions would accomplish the goal of "Help family adjust to the diagnosis"?

    a.

    b.

    c.

    d.

    e.

    f.

3. Identify a nursing diagnosis that addresses growth and development of the chronically ill child.

G. Experiential Exercise: Care for a child who has a terminal illness and his family.
1. What nursing goals would accomplish the nursing diagnosis of "Altered growth and development related to terminal illness and/or impending death"?
   a.

   b.

   c.

2. What evaluation data would reflect the meeting of the goal "Support child during terminal phase"?
   a.

   b.

V. Suggested Readings

Burns CE, Madian N: Experiences with a support group for grandparents of children with disabilities, Pediatr Nurs 18(1):17-21, 1992.

The authors present a review of the literature and, as an outcome of the support group, identify issues not previously discussed in the grandparenting literature. The support group was initiated as a means of providing support that might enhance the grandparents' coping so that they could in turn support the parents of the child with a disability. The support group was effective in achieving this goal, and also in allowing grandparents of handicapped children to help each other. The authors outline how to form a support group and how nurses can conduct meetings to accomplish the group's goals. An interesting and useful article.

Hogan NS, Balk DE: Adolescent reactions to sibling death: perceptions of mothers, fathers, and teenagers, Nurs Res 39(2):103-106, 1990.

These authors interviewed the mother, father, and one teenager from each family in which a child had died. The surprising results suggest that the father's observations and perceptions about the bereavement of their adolescent was much more congruent with those of the bereaved adolescent than were those of the mother of the same adolescent. Nurses must therefore recognize the complex dynamics related to bereavement and must assess the family carefully to intervene effectively.

Meeropol E: Parental needs assessment: a design for clinical nurse specialist practice, Pediatr Nurs 17(5):456-458, 1991.

The author incorporates a review of the literature on children with chronic illness or disability and their families. In this study parents of children with orthopedic illness or disability were asked to identify their needs and their children's needs for education and support. The most commonly identified needs were (1) information on diagnosis and treatment in the context of development, and (2) information on sexuality. Clinical nurse specialists could use the parental responses to shape their practices.

Miles A: Caring for families when a child dies, Pediatr Nurs 16(4):346-347, 1990.

The author, a minister at a children's hospital, offers personal insights to nurses caring for dying children. He offers suggestions on how to provide spiritual support to the families of the dead child.

Selekman J, McIlvain-Simpson G: Sex and sexuality for the adolescent with a chronic condition, Pediatr Nurs 17(6)535-538, 1991.

The authors explore the sexuality needs of the adolescent with a chronic condition and propose guidelines for assessment and intervention by nurses to assist the client to meet these needs.

Chapter 19
Impact of Cognitive or Sensory Impairment on the Child and Family

I. Chapter Overview

Chapter 19 introduces nursing considerations essential to the care of the child with a cognitive impairment or a sensory or communication disorder. Since these deficits pose a special threat to the child's developmental potential, it is important for students to understand the care of children with these types of disorders. At the completion of this chapter, the student should know the etiologies, detection methods, and management of cognitive impairments and sensory and communication disorders. This knowledge will enable the student to develop nursing strategies that will promote optimum realization of the child's potential.

II. Learning Objectives

Upon completion of this chapter, it is expected that the student will be able to:

1. Define the classifications of mental retardation.

2. Outline nursing interventions for the child with cognitive impairment that promote optimum development, including during hospitalization.

3. Identify the major biologic and cognitive characteristics of the child with Down syndrome.

4. Outline nursing interventions for the child with Down syndrome.

5. Identify the major characteristics associated with fragile X syndrome.

6. List the general classifications of hearing impairment and the effect on speech.

7. Outline nursing interventions for the child with hearing impairment, including during hospitalization.

8. List the common types of visual disorders in children.

9. Outline nursing interventions for the child with visual impairment, including during hospitalization.

10. Outline nursing intervention for the child with retinoblastoma.

III. Review of Essential Concepts

1. _____ is the most common developmental disability in the United States.

2. Define mental retardation.

3. Why is the term adaptive behavior a critical component of the definition of mental retardation?

4. When is a diagnosis of cognitive impairment usually made?

5. The diagnosis and classification of mental retardation is based on _____ _____.

6. Identify the four causes of severe mental retardation.
   a.

   b.

   c.

   d.

7. Identify nine prenatal, perinatal, and postnatal causes of mental retardation.
   a.

   b.

   c.

   d.

   e.

   f.

   g.

   h.

   i.

8. Describe the Education of the Handicapped Act, (PL 99-457).

9. What two principles should guide the nurse when teaching self-help skills?
   a.

   b.

10. Toys are selected for their _____.
11. _____ is a major consideration in selecting recreational and exercise activities.
12. _____ is the most common chromosomal abnormality of a generalized syndrome.
13. Approximately 95% of all cases of Down syndrome are attributable to an extra _____ chromosome.
14. How is the presence of Down syndrome confirmed?

15. ___ Children with Down syndrome usually have a normal intelligence level. (true or false)
16. What factor contributes to the development of respiratory difficulties in children with Down syndrome?

17. Differentiate among the following terms:
    a. Hearing impaired–

    b. Deaf–

    c. Hard-of-hearing–

18. List the causes of hearing impairment.
    a.

    b.

    c.

    d.

    e.

    f.

    g.

h.

i.

19. Match the following types of hearing losses with their defining characteristics. (Answers may be used more than once.)
  a. _____ conductive
  b. _____ sensorineural
  c. _____ mixed conductive-sensorineural
  d. _____ central auditory imperception
  1) most frequently occurs as the result of recurrent otitis media
  2) involves damage to the inner ear structures and/or the auditory nerve
  3) results from interference with transmission of sound in the middle ear and along neural pathways
  4) most common of all types of hearing loss
  5) deficits are divided into organic or functional losses
  6) hearing is improved with the use of a hearing aid
  7) most common causes are congenital defects of inner ear structures, or consequences of acquired conditions
  8) refers to all hearing losses that do not demonstrate defects in the conductive or sensorineural structures
  9) results in distortion of sound and problems of discrimination
  10) results from interference in transmission of sound to the middle ear
  11) also referred to as perceptive loss or nerve deafness

20. Differentiate among the following terms used to describe receptive-expressive disorders:
  a. Aphasia–

  b. Agnosia–

  c. Dysacusis–

21. How is hearing impairment described?

22. Hearing impairment is expressed in terms of _____, a unit of loudness.

23. One of the most common problems with hearing aids is _____ , an annoying whistling sound usually caused by improper fit of the ear mold.

24. When is an individual considered to be legally blind?

25. _____ are the most common causes of visual impairment.

26. Define the term *refractive errors*.

27. ___ Refractive errors are evaluated by testing visual acuity. (true or false)

28. Match the following types of refractive errors with their defining characteristics.
  a. _____ myopia
  b. _____ hyperopia
  c. _____ anisometropia
  d. _____ astigmatism
  1) also referred to as farsightedness
  2) also referred to as nearsightedness
  3) refers to unequal curvatures in the cornea or lens so that light rays are bent in different directions, producing a blurred image
  4) refers to the ability to see objects clearly at close range but not at a distance
  5) refers to a difference of refractive strength in each eye
  6) correction involves the use of specially ground lenses
  7) refers to the ability to see objects clearly at a distance
  8) correction involves the use of biconcave lenses
  9) treated with corrective lenses to improve vision in each eye so they work as a unit
  10) correction involves the use of convex lenses
  11) child often squints in an attempt to try to correct the defect

29. Define a*mblyopia*.

30. What is the most effective method for treating amblyopia?

31. _____ refers to malalignment of the eyes.

32. What occurs when there is a malalignment of the eyes?

33. The following definition of a type of strabismus is properly termed _____: "inward deviation of the eye."

34. Define the following terms:
  a. Cataract–

  b. Glaucoma–

35. Why are mobility and locomotion skills typically delayed in blind children?

36. What is the most traumatic sensory impairment?

37. Describe the effects that auditory and visual impairments have on the child's development.

38. _____ is a rare congenital malignant tumor.

39. The overall prognosis for retinoblastoma is approximately _____.

IV. Application, Analysis, and Synthesis of Essential Concepts

A. Experiential Exercise: Spend a day in an early intervention unit to observe the various methods used in the management of the child with cognitive impairment.

1. The major intervention for the prevention of mental retardation is _____ for the small premature infant and other high-risk newborns.

2. What is the major nursing goal of caring for children with mental retardation?

3. What must the nurse assess before teaching a child with subnormal intelligence?

4. What areas should the nurse assess when a child with cognitive impairment is hospitalized?
  a.

  b.

  c.

  d.

  e.

5. Identify five nursing interventions that should be used when caring for a hospitalized child who is cognitively impaired.
  a.

  b.

  c.

  d.

  e.

B. Experiential Exercise: Interview the parents of a child with Down syndrome to identify the major management problems related to this disorder. Answer the following questions and include specific responses to illustrate these concepts.

1. Briefly describe the following outstanding features of Down syndrome:
  a. Intelligence—

  b. Growth and sexual development—

  c. Congenital anomalies—

d. Sensory problems—

b. Detection of hearing loss—

3. What areas should the nurse assess when evaluating a child for a possible hearing loss?
   a. Infancy—

e. Other physical disorders—

b. Childhood—

2. What is the nurse's role when parents are informed of a diagnosis of Down syndrome in their child?
   a.

   b.

   c.

   d.

   e.

4. What type of speech is seen most often in children with a hearing impairment?
   a. mild—

   b. severe—

5. Why is it especially difficult to teach a deaf child to speak?

C. Experiential Exercise: Spend a day in a hearing clinic to observe testing, evaluation, and treatment modalities for the child with a hearing impairment. Answer the following questions and include specific examples to illustrate these concepts.
   1. Why is the hearing-impaired child at a great disadvantage for developing social relationships?

6. Identify the nursing goals that would relate to the nursing diagnosis of "Altered growth and development related to defective communication."
   a.

   b.

   c.

2. For each of the following nursing goals, list at least three nursing interventions that would be used when caring for a child with a hearing impairment and his family.
   a. Prevention of hearing loss—

D. Experiential Exercise: Spend a morning in a vision clinic to observe testing, evaluation, and treatment modalities for the child with a visual impairment. Answer the following questions and include specific examples to illustrate these concepts.
   1. Identify five nursing goals for care of the child with visual impairment and her family.
      a.

b.

c.

d.

e.

2. What instructions regarding preservation of sight should be incorporated into a preventive health teaching plan for parents?
   a.

   b.

   c.

   d.

   e.

3. When counseling the parents of an infant who is blind, what interventions would accomplish the goal of "promoting parent-child attachment"?
   a.

   b.

   c.

   d.

   e.

   f.

E. Clinical Situation: Thomas Block, age 17 months, is admitted for treatment of a retinoblastoma.
   1. The three nursing goals for the nursing care of Thomas are:
      a.

      b.

      c.

   2. List at least one nursing intervention that would accomplish each of these nursing goals.
      a.

b.

c.

V. Suggested Readings

American Academy of Pediatrics, Committee on Bioethics: Sterilization of women who are mentally handicapped, Pediatrics 85(5):868-871, 1990.

> The Committee on Bioethics concurred with the statement of the American College of Obstetricians and Gynecologists on the sterilization of mentally handicapped women (1988). The pediatricians on this committee went on to state four facets of their position.

Badger TA, Jones E: Deaf and hearing children's conceptions of body interior, Pediatr Nurs 16(2):201-205, 1990.

> This study, which involved 80 deaf children and 190 hearing children ages 5 to 15 years, was undertaken to determine if deaf and hearing children differ in their conceptions of the body interior and to examine children's conceptions of their internal bodies at three different cognitive stages. Results revealed that three groups knew significantly fewer body parts than the hearing children. Empirical support for Crider's development theory of how conceptions of the body interior develop was a secondary result of this study.

Harrison LL: Minimizing barriers when teaching hearing-impaired clients, MCN 15(2):113, 1990.

> This author discusses methods by which nurses can decrease barriers and facilitate communication with hearing-impaired clients. To enable nurses to ensure that the health education needs of deaf clients are met, the author suggests methods of communication and use of an interpreter certified in American Sign Language.

Schraeder BD, McEvoy-Shields K: Visual acuity, binocular vision, and other ocular muscle balance in VLBW children, Pediatr Nurs 17(1):30-33, 1991.

> In this study, 34 very low-birth-weight (VLBW) 6-year olds and 31 normal-birth-weight (NBW) 6-year-olds were assessed for visual acuity, binocular vision, and ocular

muscle balance. Significantly more of the children in the VLBW group failed the test of binocular vision and ocular muscle balance. Failure in tests was associated with a higher number of days on mechanical ventilation and a higher number of days in the intensive care nursery during the first months of life.

The implications for pediatric nurses is that all VLBW children should have their vision assessed periodically. Parents must be educated to the need for visual follow-up and educated about the possible impact of vision on problems in learning.

Chapter 20

Reaction of the Child and Family to Illness and Hospitalization

I. Chapter Overview

Chapter 20 provides an overview of how children of various ages react to illness and hospitalization. Since children are extremely vulnerable to the stress of such experiences, it is important to understand their reactions. Children respond to these stressors in a manner consistent with their developmental level. A child's illness and hospitalization also have a profound effect on the family unit. At the completion of this chapter, the student will be aware of how the child and his family react to the stress of illness and hospitalization and will be able to intervene to lessen the trauma of these experiences.

II. Learning Objectives

Upon completion of this chapter, it is expected that the student will be able to:

1. Identify the stressors of illness and hospitalization for children during each developmental stage.

2. Outline nursing interventions that prevent or minimize the stress of separation during hospitalization.

3. List the procedures for admitting a child to the hospital.

4. Outline nursing interventions that minimize the stress of loss of control during hospitalization.

5. Outline nursing interventions that minimize the fear of bodily injury during hospitalization.

6. Describe methods of assessing and managing pain in children.

7. Outline nursing interventions that support parents and siblings during a child's illness and hospitalization.

8. Describe nursing interventions needed when children are admitted to special units.

III. Review of Essential Concepts

1. What five factors affect the child's reaction to the stress of hospitalization?
    a.

    b.

    c.

    d.

    e.

2. From middle infancy through preschool years _____ is the major stressor related to hospitalization.

3. The three phases in the crisis of separation are _____, _____, and _____.

4. Adolescents experience the stress of separation primarily from their _____ rather than their family.

5. The three major areas in which children

experience loss of control are _____
_____, _____ or
_____, and _____.

6. The needs of children vary with age. Identify which age group the following responses to loss of control exemplify by placing the appropriate letter in the preceding blank.
   a. ___ They strive for autonomy, react with negativism to any physical restriction.
   b. ___ The same feelings that make them feel omnipotent also make them feel out of control.
   c. ___ Explanations are understood only in terms of real events.
   d. ___ Their initial reaction to dependency is negativism and aggression.
   e. ___ They respond with depression, hostility, and frustration to physical restrictions.
   f. ___ They often voluntarily isolate themselves from age-mates until they can compete on an equal basis.
   g. ___ Altering of routine and ritual results in regression.
   h. ___ Any threat to their sense of identity results in a loss of control.
   i. ___ They are particularly vulnerable to feelings of loss of control because they are striving for independence and productivity.
   j. ___ They perceive illness or hospitalization as punishment for real or imagined misdeeds.
      1) toddlers
      2) preschoolers
      3) school-age children
      4) adolescents
7. Infants less than _____ of age appear to have no memory of previous painful experiences.
8. Identify each of the following statements regarding bodily injury and pain in children as true or false.
   a. ___ Neonates' general reaction to painful stimuli is body movement associated with brief loud crying.
   b. ___ Toddlers are able to describe the type or intensity of the pain.
   c. ___ Preschoolers' primary reaction to the stress of pain and fear is aggression.
   d. ___ Distraction is an effective intervention for pain in infants.
   e. ___ School-age children use passive methods of dealing with pain.
   f. ___ Behaviors indicating pain in the toddler are grimacing, clinching teeth or lips, opening eyes wide, rocking, rubbing, and aggressiveness.
   g. ___ Adolescents react to pain with resistance and aggression.
9. List the individual risk factors that increase the child's vulnerability to the stresses of hospitalization.
   a.
   b.
   c.
   d.
   e.
   f.
10. ____ Infants and children are medicated appropriately for pain (true or false)
11. An operational definition of pain that is useful in clinical practice is:

12. Identify the fallacies or myths regarding pain relief in children:
   a.

   b.

   c.

   d.

   e.

   f.

13. QUESTT is an approach to pain assessment in children. Define this term.
   a. Q =

   b. U =

   c. E =

   d. S =

   e. T =

   f. T =

14. The seven scales that are appropriate to assess pain in children are:
   a.

   b.

   c.

   d.

   e.

f.

g.

15. Programs to prepare the child and his family for the hospitalization experience are based on what principle?

16. Identify which of the following nursing goals are appropriate to decrease the effects of bodily injury and pain in children. (Mark C before correct goals and X before incorrect goals.)
    a. ___ Preparation for painful procedures decreases fear.
    b. ___ Children should be encouraged to express pain.
    c. ___ Procedures should be explained at the child's cognitive level.
    d. ___ Ensure pain relief by administering medication on a p.r.n. basis.

17. A significant advance in the administration of intravenous analgesics is the use of
_____.

18. The major side effect from opioid medication is _____.

19. Play is the _____ of children.

20. Nursing interventions should focus on maximizing the potential benefit of the hospitalization experience by fostering _____; providing _____; promoting _____; and providing _____.

21. Parents respond to the illness and hospitalization of their child in a fairly consistent manner. What are the stages of reaction?
    a.

    b.

    c.

    d.

22. The siblings of the hospitalized child may react with feelings of:

23. Admission to an _____ room increases all the stressors typically associated with hospitalization.

24. Stressors for the child and family when in the neonatal or pediatric ICU can be grouped into four categories:
    a.

    b.

    c.

    d.

IV. Application, Analysis, and Synthesis of Essential Concepts

A. Clinical Situation: Ronik, age 2 years, was admitted to the pediatric unit with a diagnosis of meningitis. When Ronik's parents briefly left the room, Ronik began to shake the bars of the crib, to scream and cry loudly, and refuse attention from the nurse.
   1. When the nurse assesses Ronik's behavior, she knows it is characteristic of the _____ stage of separation.
   2. List at least one appropriate intervention to deal with Ronik's behavior.

B. Clinical Situation: Amy, 2 years old, was admitted to the pediatric unit for evaluation and treatment of a urinary tract infection. Both Amy and her parents appear anxious.
   1. Identify at least three nursing interventions to accomplish the nursing goal of minimizing the effects of separation for Amy.
      a.

      b.

      c.

   2. Identify at least two nursing interventions to accomplish the nursing goal of minimizing the effects of loss of control.
      a.

      b.

C. Clinical Situation: Roberto, age 4 years, is admitted to the pediatric unit with a diagnosis of gastroenteritis.

1. List the primary nursing goals for support of the family of a hospitalized child.

   a.

   b.

   c.

   d.

2. List at least three nursing interventions to accomplish the nursing goal of supporting the parents of the hospitalized child.

   a.

   b.

   c.

   d.

   e.

3. List at least three nursing interventions to accomplish the nursing goal of promoting and fostering positive family relationships.

   a.

   b.

   c.

   d.

4. Roberto's mother asks you, the nurse, for advice on what toys she should bring to her child. With consideration for developmental needs and for safety, what types of toys would you recommend?

D. Clinical Situation: Manuel, age 6 years, is being admitted to the pediatric unit with a complaint of abdominal pain.

1. What steps (interventions) should the nurse follow when admitting Manuel to the unit?

   a.

   b.

   c.

2. What steps (interventions) should the nurse follow to establish a trusting relationship with the child?

   a.

   b.

   c.

   d.

   e.

   f.

   g.

V. Suggested Readings

Greenberg LA: Teaching children who are learning-disabled about illness and hospitalization, MCN 16(5):260-263, 1991.

> A contemporary and comprehensive exploration of this topic. Aspects covered include definition of learning disabilities and definition and explanation of different types of learners (auditory learner, visual learner, tactile learner, integrative processing disability, short and/or long-term memory disability, language disability, and motor disability). A very helpful and detailed discussion of interventions to accommodate a disability in a child is presented. An interesting aspect of this article is its list of myths and facts concerning disabilities. The interventions can be particularly helpful to the pediatric nurse.

Grimm DL, Pefley PT: Opening doors for the child "inside," Pediatr Nurs 16(4):368-369, 1990.

> Two pediatric nurses report on an opportunity to collaborate on a project that offered songs,

stories, and laughter to help children talk about the many emotional issues raised during hospitalization.

Gureno MA, Reisinger CL: Patient-controlled analgesia for the young pediatric patient, Pediatr Nurs 17(3):252-254, 1991.

A collaborative effort at St. Luke's Hospital in Cedar Rapids sought to improve pain control in young pediatric patients. This effort resulted in new policies and a change in pain management practice. Patient-controlled analgesia was identified as a successful method of pain control for children as young as 3 years old.

Kennedy CM, and others: A nursing tool to assess children upon hospital admission, MCN 16(2):78-82, 1991.

The authors report on a pediatric admission assessment tool developed at St. Louis Children's Hospital in 1987. This tool can help pediatric nurses effectively identify, communicate, and alleviate the needs of hospitalized children and their families.

Morrison RA: Update on sickle cell disease: incidence of addiction and choice of opioid in pain management, Pediatr Nurs 17(5):503, 1991.

Two important concerns in pain management of children with sickle cell disease—addiction and choice of drug—are reviewed. The author bases her conclusions on 13 years of experience and more than 630 pediatric patients with pain due to this disease. The author contends that addiction does not have an increased incidence in this population. The author also emphasizes contraindication of the use of meperidine with sickle cell clients.

Vessey JA, and others: Iatrogenic developmental effects of pediatric intensive care, Pediatr Nurs 17(3):229-232, 1991.

This article identifies iatrogenic factors that interfere with the achievement of normal developmental milestones in critically ill children in pediatric intensive care environments. Knowledge of these factors can help the nurse develop the skills and sensitivity to meet the complex needs of these children and their families.

Chapter 21
Pediatric Variations of Nursing Interventions

I. Chapter Overview

Chapter 21 provides an overview of the common variations of nursing procedures that must be implemented when working with children. Since children differ from adults in the areas of biologic, cognitive, and emotional function and response, it is important for the student to understand how nursing practice must be altered to meet the special needs of the pediatric patient. Small children who are hospitalized are separated from their usual environment and do not possess the capacity for abstract thinking and reasoning, which has ramifications both for compliance and for safety. At the completion of this chapter the student should have the theoretical basis to be able to safely implement nursing procedures specific to the pediatric population.

II. Learning Objectives

Upon completion of this chapter, it is expected that the student will be able to:

1. Identify the instances in which informed consent is required and in which minors may be considered emancipated.

2. Formulate general guidelines for preparing children for procedures, including surgery.

3. Implement uses of play in therapeutic procedures.

4. List general strategies for enhancing compliance in children and families.

5. Outline general hygiene and care procedures for hospitalized children.

6. Implement feeding techniques that encourage food and fluid intake.

7. Describe methods of reducing temperature in a child with fever or hyperthermia.

8. Describe systems that can be used for infection control.

9. Describe safe methods of administering oral, parenteral, rectal, optic, otic, and nasal medications to children.

10. Identify nursing responsibilities in maintaining fluid balance.

11. Demonstrate correct procedure for postural drainage and tracheostomy care.

12. Describe the procedures involved in providing nutrition via gavage, gastrostomy, and parenteral routes.

13. Describe the procedure involved in administering an enema and ostomy care to children.

III. Review of Essential Concepts

1. What is informed consent?

2. Three conditions must be met for an informed consent to be valid. What are they?
   a.

   b.

   c.

3. In relation to informed consent the nurse should know the state law regarding an emancipated or mature minor, and the age of majority. Define the following:
   a. Emancipated minor—

   b. Mature minor—

4. Children, regardless of their age require _____ to minimize the fear and discomfort experienced during procedures.

5. When preparing children for procedures, the nurse must consider which factors to individualize the preparation?
   a.

   b.

   c.

   d.

   e.

6. ___ Procedures should be performed in the child's room whenever possible. (true or false)

7. What four areas of supportive care should the nurse consider before a procedure?
   a.

   b.

   c.

   d.

8. Play can be used as part of nursing care. Play can be used to:
   a.

   b.

   c.

9. The six stress points before and after surgery that can cause anxiety are:
   a.

   b.

   c.

   d.

   e.

   f.

10. Research indicates that a child may receive clear liquids up to _____ hours before surgery without risk of aspiration.

11. The definition of compliance is:

12. When assessing compliance, the nurse would use a combination of two measurement techniques. List the techniques used to measure compliance.
    a.

    b.

    c.

    d.

    e.

    f.

    g.

13. Strategies to enhance compliance are grouped into three categories. They are:
    a.

    b.

    c.

14. To care for their hair properly, black children need to have a comb with _____ _____ and a jar of _____.

15. If diarrhea is present, high carbohydrate liquids are _____ because they may aggravate the diarrhea by an _____ effect.

16. Evidence of lack of readiness to advance the diet is:

a.

b.

c.

d.

e.

17. One of the most common symptoms of illness in children is _____.

18. Match the following terms regarding body temperature with their definitions.
___ set point
___ fever
___ hyperthermia
  a. an elevation in set point such that body temperature is regulated at a higher level
  b. body temperature exceeds set point
  c. the temperature around which body temperature is regulated

19. In treating fever, the most effective intervention is the use of _____ to lower the set point.

20. Shivering will _____ (increase, decrease) the body temperature.

21. The two types of isolation precautions are:

a.

b.

22. _____ is the most critical infection control practice.

23. Discipline is necessary to ensure a child's safety in the hospital. A useful discipline technique is the _____.

24. The method of transporting children safely is determined by their:

a.

b.

c.

25. _____ are never used as a punishment or as a substitute for observation.

26. Urine obtained from disposable diapers can be tested accurately for _____.

27. The midstream urine specimen procedure must be modified for the child who cannot void on command. What modification is necessary?

28. _____ may be used to increase the adhesion of the 24-hour collecting bag.

29. The method most used to determine accurate drug dosage for a child is _____ _____.

30. The only safe method for identifying a child is to _____.

31. What are the preferred sites for injections in infants and small children?

a.

b.

32. What are the factors the nurse must consider when administering intravenous drugs to infants and children?

a.

b.

c.

d.

e.

f.

g.

33. Differentiate between the following methods of administering medications through IV tubing in the child.

a. Direct technique–

b. Retrograde technique–

34. _____ provide for long-term intravenous administration of drugs.

35. Identify the type of venous access devices currently available.

   a.

   b.

   c.

36. To prevent the problem of evaporative losses and leakage of excreta, diapers should be weighed _____
_____.

37. Intravenous infusion pumps are widely used in pediatrics because:

38. The organs most vulnerable to damage from excessive oxygenation are the _____ and the _____.

39. Noninvasive methods of determining oxygen saturation are:

   a.

   b.

40. List the advantages of administering medication by aerosol therapy.

   a.

   b.

   c.

41. ___ Bronchial drainage is more effective immediately after aerosol therapy. (true or false)

42. CPT = _____.

43. Air or gas delivered directly to the trachea must be _____.

44. Signs of impending occlusion of a tracheostomy are:

45. When suctioning the tracheostomy, the nurse must advance the catheter to the premeasured depth of no more than _____ beyond the tube.

46. How often is the tracheostomy suctioned?

47. Measurement of the nasogastric or orogastric tube insertion distance has been done by two standard methods. What new method is promising to be more accurate?

48. For children who will be on long-term gastrostomy feeding, a skin level device called the _____ or _____ offers several advantages when compared with the conventional gastrostomy tube.

49. Total parenteral nutrition (TPN), is also known as _____ or _____.

50. Plain water is not used in an enema for children because, being hypotonic, it can cause _____.

51. Fleet's enema is not recommended for children. What are the possible complications of this form of enema?

   a.

   b.

52. A major nursing responsibility in the care of ostomies is to protect the _____ from breakdown.

IV. Application, Analysis, and Synthesis of Essential Concepts

A. Clinical Situation: Murray, 5 years old, is scheduled to have a lumbar puncture performed.

   1. What interventions would the nurse institute to accomplish the nursing goal of completing needed procedures safely and with a minimum of stress for the child? List them.

   a.

   b.

   c.

   d.

   e.

B. Clinical Situation: Franklin, age 5 years, is admitted to the unit for surgery.

1. What nursing goals would address the nursing diagnosis of "High risk for injury related to surgical procedure, anesthesia" for Franklin?

   a.

   b.

   c.

   d.

   e.

   f.

2. What interventions would achieve the goal of increasing Franklin's sense of security?

   a.

   b.

   c.

3. What evaluative data would you expect if the nursing goal of "Promote adequate hydration" was accomplished postoperatively?

   a.

   b.

C. Clinical Situation: Juan is admitted with a diagnosis of meningitis and has a fever of 103° F.

1. How and when would you evaluate whether your intervention of administration of an antipyretic is effective?

2. What interventions on the environment will help reduce Juan's fever?

3. To ensure Juan's safety, you would always make sure the _____ are in the "up" position.

D. Clinical Situation: Maia, age 4 years, is being discharged after hospitalization for pneumonia.

1. What parameters of care would you teach to her parents to enable them to care for Maia at home?

   a.

   b.

   c.

   d.

   e.

2. What would you tell these parents regarding selection of toys for play?

E. Clinical Situation: Jonathan, age 1 year, needs to have both legs restrained to protect the surgical site and the catheter in his penis.

1. What is the rationale for each of the following interventions?

   a. Applying a clove hitch restraint to Jonathan's extremities.

   b. Removing Jonathan's restraints every 2 hours.

F. Experiential Exercise: Spend a morning on a pediatric floor and survey the type, route, amount, and method of administration of the medications being provided to the children.

1. When administering an oral medication, the nurse should try to avoid mixing it with food or liquid. If she must mix it, what guidelines (interventions) should she follow? Give a rationale for each guideline.

   a.

   b.

G. Clinical Situation: Mariano, age 6 months, is a patient on the pediatric unit. He was admitted to the unit in severe respiratory distress. He was placed in a mist tent in 30% oxygen.

1. List the interventions that can be used to lessen Mariano's fear of the mist tent.

   a.

   b.

   c.

   d.

2. What is the rationale for performing chest physiotherapy before meals or 1 to 2 hours after feeding?

3. How would the nurse evaluate whether the chest physiotherapy was successful in removing excess fluid?

H. Clinical Situation: Raoul, age 11 months, is a patient on the pediatric unit. He was admitted to the unit in respiratory failure and a tracheostomy was performed.
   1. List the nursing interventions used to care for Raoul's tracheostomy.
      a.

      b.

      c.

      d.

      e.

      f.

   2. What would the nurse assess in Raoul to determine that his lungs need to be suctioned?

I. Clinical Situation: Debra, 1 day old, is admitted to the pediatric floor for medical evaluation. She has a weak suck reflex and cannot drink from a bottle adequately. She is being fed 1 ounce of Enfamil via gavage every 3 hours.
   1. Give a rationale for each of the following interventions the nurse would perform when feeding Debra via gavage.
      a. Insert feeding tube through mouth—

      b. When checking placement of feeding tube, return aspirated contents to stomach—

      c. Secure feeding tube to cheek, not forehead—

   d. Flush indwelling feeding tube with 1 ml sterile water—

   e. Position Debra on right side or abdomen after feedings—

2. Before inserting formula in the feeding tube, the nurse assesses whether the tube is correctly positioned in the stomach by:
   a.

   b.

3. What interventions regarding gavage feeding are validated by these rationales?
   a. Refeed to prevent electrolyte imbalance—

   b. So that sucking is associated with feeding—

V. **Suggested Readings**

Beecroft PC, Redick SA: Intramuscular injection practices of pediatric nurses: site selection, Nurse Educator 15(4):23-27, 1990.

   The authors review relevant literature and discuss study findings related to site description, boundaries, site selection, and complications. Implications for nurse educators are presented.

Bender LH, and others: Postoperative patient-controlled analgesia in children, Pediatr Nurs 16(6):549-554, 1990.

   Patient-controlled analgesia (PCA) has proven to be effective in adult clients. The authors discuss the use of PCA with children who have had surgery. The discussion highlights the following aspects of this treatment: assessment and management of pain in children and adolescents, use of patient-controlled analgesia, patient selection for PCA use, patient teaching, and nursing care. This article is a must for pediatric nurses caring for surgical clients.

Bockus S: Troubleshooting your tube feedings, Am Nurs 91(5):24-28, 1991.

> The author discusses the advantages and disadvantages of three tube-feeding routes in the areas of placement, residuals, aspiration, gastrointestinal complications, fluid and electrolyte imbalance, and managing patient and tube. This is an ANA-approved continuing education offering.

Holder C, Alexander J: A new and improved guide to IV therapy, Am Nurs 90(2):43-47, 1990.

> A detailed chart based on research instructs the nurse on how to flush, the frequency of flush, changes of dressing, drawing of blood, changing of caps, the removal of lines, and troubleshooting for 12 frequently used intravenous catheters.

Kandt KA: An implantable venous access device for children, MCN 16(2):88-91, 1991.

> The pros and cons of using the implantable venous access device (IVAD) in children are discussed. Guidelines for nursing management of the device and a complete nursing care plan are presented.

Lybrand M, and others: Periodic comparisons of specific gravity using urine from a diaper and collecting bag, MCN 15(4):238-239, 1990.

> This study demonstrates that the specific gravity of urine collected from a diaper can be reliably assessed for up to two hours after a neonate voids.

Swift RR: Rational management of a child's acute fever, MCN 15(2):82-85, 1990.

> The author discusses the potential benefits and harm of acute fever and the benefits and risks of antipyretic medication. Implications for patient education are included.

Chapter 22

The Child with Respiratory Dysfunction

I. Chapter Overview

Chapter 22 introduces nursing considerations essential to the care of the child experiencing respiratory dysfunction. Because some of the most common problems in the pediatric age group are related to disturbed respiratory function, and respiratory failure is the primary cause of morbidity in the newborn period, it is important for the student to gain an understanding of the care of children with these types of disorders. The conditions discussed in this chapter impair the exchange of oxygen and/or carbon dioxide and are often more serious in young children. At the completion of this chapter, the student will be able to formulate nursing goals and identify nursing responsibilities to help the child and his family effectively cope with the physical, emotional, and psychosocial stressors imposed by an alteration in respiratory function.

II. Learning Objectives

Upon completion of this chapter, it is expected that the student will be able to:

1. Identify the significant differences between the respiratory tract of the infant or young child and that of the adult.

2. Contrast the effects of various respiratory infections observed in infants and children.

3. Describe the postoperative nursing care of the child with a tonsillectomy.

4. Outline a nursing plan for a child with croup.

5. Outline a nursing care plan for a child with acute otitis media.

6. Demonstrate an understanding of the ways in which inhalation of noninfectious irritants produces pulmonary dysfunction.

7. Describe the ways in which the various therapeutic measures relieve the symptoms of asthma.

8. Outline a plan for teaching home care for the child with bronchial asthma.

9. Describe the physiologic effects of cystic fibrosis on the gastrointestinal and pulmonary systems.

10. Outline a plan of care for the child with cystic fibrosis.

11. List the major signs of respiratory distress in infants and children.

III. Review of Essential Concepts

1. _____ is the chief cause of morbidity in the neonatal period.

2. What are the factors that influence the incidence and severity of respiratory infections?

    a.

    b.

c.

d.

e.

f.

g.

3. The largest percentage of infections is caused by _____.
4. Explain why size is a significant variable in respiratory infection of the child.

5. Infants and young children develop generalized signs and symptoms as well as local symptoms within respiratory infection. Identify the following statements as true or false.
   a. ___ Newborns may not develop a fever even with severe infections.
   b. ___ The 6-month- to 3-year-old will develop fever even with a mild respiratory illness.
   c. ___ Febrile convulsions occur with a gradual rise in temperature.
   d. ___ Meningeal signs without infection of the meninges may be present in small children who have an abrupt onset of fever.
   e. ___ Vomiting is uncommon with respiratory infection.
   f. ___ Diarrhea may accompany respiratory infection.
   g. ___ Abdominal pain is an uncommon complaint in small children with a respiratory infection.
   h. ___ Respiratory illness causes difficulty with feeding because of nasal blockage.
6. _____ may be instilled to clear nasal passages and promote feeding.
7. What is the rationale for use of warm or cool mist?

8. What is a quick method of producing humidification?

9. The therapy for nasopharyngitis is primarily _____.
10. If a child is coughing but has a profuse nasal discharge, potent antitussives are avoided. Why?

11. Acute pharyngitis of bacterial origin is usually caused by _____.
12. A _____ must be done to differentiate between a viral and hemolytic streptococcal infection.
13. The recommended treatment for a streptococcal sore throat is:

14. The function of the tonsils is:

15. The _____ are those removed during a tonsillectomy.
16. The pharyngeal tonsils are also known as the _____.
17. The clinical manifestations of tonsillitis are primarily caused by _____. Because of swelling, the child has difficulty _____ and _____.
18. Because of the proximity of the adenoids to the eustachian tubes, adenoids cause:

19. The indication for the tonsillectomy and adenoidectomy procedure is controversial. A tonsillectomy is recommended when:
   a.

   An adenoidectomy is recommended when:
   b.

20. Tonsils should not be removed until after 3 or 4 years of age. Why?
   a.

   b.

21. Postoperative nursing assessment of a tonsillectomy and adenoidectomy includes:

22. Analgesics following a tonsillectomy and adenoidectomy should be administered for at least _____.

23. The major complication of a T and A is _____.

24. The terminology regarding otitis media is confusing. List the accepted definitions for the following terms:
    a. Otitis media–

    b. Acute otitis media–

    c. Otitis media with effusion–

    d. Subacute otitis media–

    e. Chronic otitis media with effusion–

25. Acute otitis media is most frequently caused by:

26. The etiology of the noninfectious type of otitis media is unknown, although this type is frequently a result of _____ _____ from the edema of allergic rhinitis or hypertrophic adenoids.

27. The principal functional consequence of prolonged middle ear pathology is _____ _____.

28. In acute otitis media otoscopy reveals an _____ _____ _____.

29. The antimicrobial of choice for initial treatment of acute otitis media is _____ or _____.

30. Following antibiotic therapy, the child should be evaluated for the effectiveness of the treatment to identify the potential complication of _____.

31. _____ are often used to treat otitis media with effusion.

32. Croup is usually described according to:

33. The most serious complication of croup is _____.

34. The major objective in medical management of laryngotracheobronchitis (LTB) is maintaining an _____ and providing for _____.

35. Why is the child with LTB placed in an atmosphere of high humidity with cool mist? State the rationale.

36. Acute epiglottitis is:

37. Epiglottitis causes a _____ epiglottis.

38. The nurse should not examine the throat of a child with suspected epiglottitis with a tongue depressor because:

39. The _____ is the causative agent of 50% to 75% of the cases of bronchiolitis.

40. The primary pathophysiologic process in bronchiolitis that causes difficulty is:

41. Pneumonia is caused by four etiologic processes: _____, _____ _____, _____, and _____ _____.

42. The etiologic agent of pneumonia is identified from:

43. The causative organism in tuberculosis is _____.

44. In the absence of positive evidence, diagnosis of tuberculosis (TB) is based on information derived from the:

45. The single most important therapeutic modality for TB is _____.

46. What are the three most commonly used drugs to treat TB?

a.

b.

c.

47. The only certain means to prevent tuberculosis is to _____ with the tubercle bacillus. Limited immunity can be produced by administration of the

_____

vaccine.

48. Small children are particularly vulnerable to aspiration of foreign bodies because:

49. Initially, a foreign body in the air passages produces:

50. Foreign bodies are usually removed by direct _____ and

_____ .

51. It is the obligation of nurses to learn two simple procedures to treat aspiration of a foreign body. The nurse should learn and teach the following techniques:_____
_____ and the _____.

52. It is important to use these techniques only when a child is truly in distress. A child who is in distress _____,
_____, and
_____ .

53. Aspiration rarely causes death from asphyxia. The irritated mucous membrane becomes a site for _____.

54. The major nursing goal regarding aspiration is aimed at _____.

55. Smoke inhalation causes two different types of injury:

a.

b.

56. Gases that are nontoxic to the airways can cause injury and death by interfering with or inhibiting cellular respiration. _____
_____ is responsible for more than half of the fatal poisonings in the United States.

57. The symptoms of carbon monoxide are secondary to tissue hypoxia and vary with the level of carboxyhemoglobin. The treatment for a suspected poisoning is the administration of _____.

58. _____ during childhood may well be the most important precursor of chronic lung disease in the adult.

59. Bronchial asthma is defined as:

60. The usual cause of asthmatic manifestations is an:

61. Identify three mechanisms that are responsible for the obstructive symptoms of asthma.

a.

b.

c.

62. _____ is the central physiologic feature in the clinical manifestations of asthma. This forces the individual to breathe at a _____
_____ .

63. Children with bronchial asthma exhibit three major symptoms during acute attacks.

a.

b.

c.

64. The overall goal of asthma management is to _____
and to minimize _____
_____ and _____
_____ morbidity and to help the child to live as normal and happy a life as possible.

65. _____ control is basic to any therapeutic plan.

66. Early recognition and treatment at the onset are important The goal of drug therapy is to _____
_____ .

67. _____
are the major therapeutic agents for the
relief of bronchospasm.
68. What are the two types of bronchodilator
drugs?
a.

b.

69. The most effective and versatile asthmatic
drugs are the _____ drugs.
70. What is the role of exercise in the management of asthma?

71. What components of physical therapy are
essential to the management of the asthmatic child?
a.

b.

c.

72. Define *status asthmaticus*.

73. The drug of choice for status asthmaticus is
_____.
74. The four principles of self-management of
asthma are:
a.

b.

c.

d.

75. Cystic fibrosis is a _____
_____.
76. Cystic fibrosis is inherited as an _____
_____.
77. The primary pathologic factor in cystic
fibrosis is:

78. _____ are present
in almost all children with cystic fibrosis
and constitute the most serious threat to
life.

79. Describe the effects of thickened secretions
on the gastrointestinal tract of the child
with cystic fibrosis.

80. The earliest manifestation of cystic fibrosis
is _____ in the newborn.
81. Owing to the large amount of undigested
food excreted, the stools of the child with
cystic fibrosis become _____
_____.
82. The diagnosis of cystic fibrosis is based on
four findings. List them.
a.

b.

c.

d.

83. The presence of a positive _____
is characteristic of cystic fibrosis.
84. The child with cystic fibrosis should be
placed on a diet that is _____
_____
_____.
85. The goal of pulmonary therapy is:

86. What three techniques are employed to
improve ventilation in the child with cystic
fibrosis?
a.

b.

c.

87. The ultimate prognosis for the child with
cystic fibrosis is determined by the degree of
_____.

IV. Application, Analysis, and Synthesis of Essential Concepts

A. Clinical Situation: Theodore, age 6 months, is
hospitalized with an acute upper respiratory
tract infection. Theodore has a fever (104° F),
rhinitis, nasal congestion, difficulty feeding,
and diarrhea.

1. List the possible nursing diagnoses for Theodore.

   a.

   b.

   c.

   d.

   e.

   f.

   g.

   h.

B. Clinical Situation: Karen, age 11 months, is seen at the pediatrician's office for a complaint of ear pain and a fever of 102° F. A diagnosis of otitis media is made.

   1. You would intervene with Karen's parents by teaching them the signs of otitis media. List the signs.

2. What interventions regarding drug therapy will accomplish the nursing goal of "prevention of complications"?

C. Clinical Situation: Peter, age 20 months, is admitted to the pediatric unit with a diagnosis of acute laryngotracheobronchitis. His symptoms on admission included fever, hoarseness, a brassy cough, pallor, rales and rhonchi, and restlessness.

   1. What would you assess to establish Peter's respiratory status and detect any impending airway obstruction?

   2. Identify the nursing goals appropriate for Peter.

      a.

      b.

      c.

      d.

      e.

      f.

   3. What is the rationale for the use of high humidity with cool mist?

D. Experiential Exercise: Spend a day on a pediatric unit and observe the children admitted for treatment of pneumonia. Differentiate among the various types of pneumonia by completing the following chart.

	Viral	Primary Atypical	Bacteria
Etiology	1.	2.	3.
Clinical Manifestations	4.	5.	6.
Therapeutic Management	7.	8.	9.

E. Experiential Exercise: Observe small children at play.
  1. List at least two of the nursing measures necessary to prevent aspiration of foreign bodies or of liquids by children.
     a.

     b.

F. Clinical Situation: Alice, a 6-year-old white female, came to the emergency room with acute respiratory distress. Her mother noted that she was well until an hour before, when she began to cough without production and "couldn't catch her breath." There is a family history of asthma (her father) and hay fever (her mother).
  1. When you take a nursing history from Alice and her mother, what are the pertinent findings that you know predispose her to asthma?

2. What signs and symptoms of an acute asthmatic attack did you assess in Alice?

3. As the attack progresses, what additional symptoms would you expect to assess?

4. Alice will be treated with epinephrine. Before administering this drug, the nurse should know the intended effects and side effects of the drug.
   a. Intended effects—

   b. Side effects—

5. What parameters would you use to assess Alice's condition?

6. What parameters would the nurse assess to recognize *status asthmaticus*?

7. List the goals that guide the nursing care plan for the child with asthma.
   a.

   b.

   c.

   d.

   e.

   f.

G. Clinical Situation: Dennis, age 3 years, is hospitalized for treatment of cystic fibrosis.
  1. List the possible nursing diagnoses that are essential to planning the nursing care of Dennis.
     a.

b.

c.

d.

e.

f.

g.

h.

i.

j.

2. What are the evaluative data that would give evidence of the attainment of the nursing goal, "help the patient expectorate sputum"?

3. Give a rationale for each of the following clinical manifestations that Dennis displays.
   a. Respiratory symptoms—

   b. Large, bulky, frothy, foul-smelling stools—

   c. Voracious appetite—

   d. Weight loss—

   e. Anemia and bruising—

4. Dennis will be going home soon, and his mother must be taught the pulmonary therapy nec-

essary for Dennis's care. You would intervene by teaching what three procedures?
   a.

   b.

   c.

H. Clinical Situation: Reggie, age 14 years, is admitted to the hospital unit with a diagnosis of suspected tuberculosis.
   1. The most important test to establish a diagnosis of tuberculosis is _____

   _____.

   2. When teaching Reggie about his drug therapy, the nurse must keep what two principles in mind?
      a.

      b.

V. Suggested Readings

Everett D: For a child with pneumonia there's no place like home, RN 90(3):85-88, 1990.

> The author gives a detailed plan of care for the nurse who cares for a child with pneumonia in the home setting. Teaching the family to assume care is also addressed.

Gomberg SM: Mistaken identity...Is it epiglottitis or croup? Pediatr Nurs 16(6):567-570, 1990.

> When a child enters the emergency room with acute respiratory distress, it is essential to determine the cause of the distress. This article contrasts the causes, diagnosis, and medical and nursing support of the client affected by each of these respiratory illnesses and the family.

Krasinski K, and others: Screening for respiratory syncytial virus and assignment to a cohort at admission to reduce nosocomial transmission, Pediatr 116(6):894-897, 1990.

> The purpose of this study was to test methods of preventing the spread of the respiratory syncytial virus to high-risk noninfected hospitalized infants and toddlers. Although handwashing is identified as the greatest deterrent to the spread of the virus, hospitalized chil-

dren continue to acquire the infection. In this study, infants and children were screened using the ELISA method to determine if they were harboring the RSV, and then they were placed in two completely separate hospital units based on the result. By segregating the infected children from the noninfected high-risk group, the transfer of the virus within the hospital was significantly reduced.

Madsen LA: Tuberculosis today, RN 90(3):44-51, 1990.

Tuberculosis has been on the rise since 1985. Resistant strains of the Mycobacterium tuberculosis bacilli have been surfacing. This article traces the pathogenesis, screening tests, diagnosis, and the most appropriate multidrug treatment for tuberculosis. The public health goal is to completely eradicate this debilitating disease. Nurses must have current knowledge of this disease to intervene quickly and appropriately.

Shartz-Engel N: Updated on theophylline for asthma in children, MCN 16(2):134, 1991.

Theophylline is the primary therapy used to treat asthma in children. This author discusses studies that have identified behavioral, academic, and sleep problems in children taking theophylline. Findings of these studies suggest that mildly or moderately asthmatic children may benefit from alternative therapies such as cromolyn.

Tizzano EF, Buchwald M: Cystic fibrosis: beyond the gene to therapy, Pediatr 120(3):337-349, 1992.

The authors present a detailed analysis of the following topics: isolation and characterization of the cystic fibrosis gene; correlation of genotype to phenotype; current status of diagnosis, prenatal testing, and screening; cystic fibrosis transmembrane regulator and the molecular basis of chloride channel dysregulation; and prospects for therapy. This is a contemporary and technical discussion of the current knowledge regarding genes and cystic fibrosis.

Chapter 23

The Child with Gastrointestinal Dysfunction

I. Chapter Overview

Chapter 23 introduces nursing considerations essential to the care of the child experiencing gastrointestinal dysfunction. Since disorders of the gastrointestinal tract are very common and constitute one of the largest categories of illnesses in infancy and childhood, it is important for the student to understand the care of children with such alterations in health. At the completion of this chapter, the student will be able to assess the child with alteration in gastrointestinal function and will be able to develop goals and responsibilities to help child and family cope with the physical, emotional, and psychosocial stress imposed by an alteration in gastrointestinal function.

II. Learning Objectives

Upon completion of this chapter, it is expected that the student will be able to:

1. Describe the characteristics of infants that affect their ability to adapt to fluid loss or gain.

2. Formulate a plan of care for the infant with acute diarrhea.

3. Formulate a plan for teaching the parents preoperative and postoperative care of a child with a cleft lip and/or palate.

4. Compare the preoperative and postoperative care of an infant with a structural defect of the gastrointestinal tract.

5. Identify nutritional therapies for a child with malabsorption syndrome.

6. Formulate a plan of care for a child with an obstructive disorder.

7. Compare and contrast the inflammatory diseases of the gastrointestinal tract.

8. Describe the cause, prevention, and nursing care of the child with hepatitis.

III. Review of Essential Concepts

1. Dehydration results when _____ _____.

2. Infants are prone to disturbance in fluid and electrolytes because they have?
   a. a decreased amount of surface area
   b. a slower metabolic rate
   c. decreased ability to handle solutes and water
   d. decreased amounts of extracellular fluid

3. ___ Sodium is the major osmotic force controlling fluid movement. (true or false)

4. A sign or symptom of isotonic dehydration is:
   a. seizures
   b. serum sodium below 130 mEq/1
   c. signs of shock
   d. increased urine output

5. How is diarrhea defined?

6. ___ Chronic diarrhea is often a result of an infectious process. (true or false)
7. A common clinical manifestation of diarrhea is:
   a. shock
   b. overhydration
   c. metabolic alkalosis
   d. dehydration
8. The most widely used test to differentiate bacterial from viral infections is determining the presence of _____.
9. Intravenous fluid therapy in mild or moderate diarrhea is directed toward:

10. Most organisms that cause gastroenteritis are spread by the _____ _____or by _____ _____.
11. ____ Rhinoviruses are the most common causes of winter diarrhea in children under the age of 2. (true or false)
12. A stool pH of less than 6 and the presence of reducing substances is suggestive of _____.
13. ___ Oral rehydration therapy (ORT) is an effective, safer, less painful, and less costly procedure than intravenous rehydration. (true or false)
14. Research shows that human milk feeding during diarrheal illness results in _____.
15. The most common causative bacterial agent of gastroenteritis in children 6 months to 10 years of age is _____.
16. _____ and _____ are the parasites that most commonly cause acute infectious diarrhea.
17. _____ is the most common cause of constipation in children between 1 and 3 years of age.
18. The primary defect in congenital megacolon is the absence of _____ _____ _____ in one segment of the colon.
19. The functional defect in aganglionic megacolon is _____ _____ _____ in the affected section of the colon.
20. _____ is performed to confirm the diagnosis of congenital megacolon.
21. The primary treatment of congenital megacolon is _____.

22. Gastroesophageal reflux (GER) is defined as:

23. Although controversial, current research recommends which positions as treatment of GER in infants?
    a.

    b.

24. List the clinical manifestations of appendicitis.
    a.

    b.

    c.

    d.

    e.

    f.

    g.

    h.

    i.

    j.

    k.

    l.

25. The site of most intense pain in appendicitis is _____ located at a point midway between the _____ _____ _____.
26. ___ Rebound tenderness is a reliable sign of appendicitis in the child. (true or false)
27. Meckel's diverticulum is defined as an _____.
28. Bleeding can occur in Meckel's diverticulum because:

29. Diagnosis of Meckel's diverticulum is usually based on _____.
30. Treatment of Meckel's diverticulum is _____.

31. The prognosis is better for which of the inflammatory bowel diseases (IBD), Crohn disease or ulcerative colitis?

32. The drug _____ has proved effective in decreasing the frequency of recurrences in patient with mild cases of IBD.

33. Surgical intervention is a more effective treatment for Crohn disease or ulcerative colitis?

34. List the clinical manifestations suggestive of peptic ulcer in children over 6 years old:

35. The objectives of therapy for children with peptic ulcers is:
  a.

  b.

  c.

  d.

36. Hepatitis is caused by at least five types of viruses. List these viruses and their abbreviations.
  a.

  b.

  c.

  d.

  e.

37. Compare the features of HAV vs. HBV by completing the following chart.

	Type A (HAV)	**Type B (HBV)**
Mode of Transmission	a.	b.
Onset	c.	d.
Immunity	e.	f.

38. What antibody or antigen is important in the diagnosis of HBV?

39. Identify whether the following statements related to hepatitis A or hepatitis B are true or false.
  a. ___ There is no specific treatment for either hepatitis A or hepatitis B.
  b. ___ Isolation is required to prevent transmission of the disease.
  c. ___ If a client has had hepatitis A he has crossover immunity to hepatitis B.
  d. ___ Immune serum globulin (ISG) is effective in preventing hepatitis A.
  e. ___ Handwashing is the single most effective measure in prevention and control of hepatitis.

40. Cirrhosis occurs as a result of _____, _____, and _____. A cirrhotic liver is _____ damaged.

41. The prognosis for infants with extrahepatic atresia is _____ and _____.

42. The major potential handicap for a child with a cleft palate is _____.

43. The immediate nursing problem in the care of the newborn with cleft lip and palate deformities is related to _____ the newborn.

44. Clinical manifestations that may indicate the presence of esophageal atresia in a newborn are:
  a.

  b.

  c.

  d.

  e.

45. List the three C's of a tracheoesophageal fistula:

46. A hernia is _____

_____

47. A hernia that cannot be reduced easily is called an _____ hernia

48. A characteristic symptom of pyloric stenosis is _____ vomiting.

49. Surgical correction of pyloric stenosis is called _____

50. Intussusception can be defined as:

51. The stool of the infant with intussusception is characteristically described as _____ _____.

52. Definitive diagnosis of intussusception is based on a _____.

53. _____ is a term applied to a long list of disorders associated with some degree of impaired digestion and/or absorption.

54. Absorptive defects include conditions in which the _____ _____ is impaired.

55. The major clinical manifestations of celiac disease are:

a.

b.

c.

d.

56. Celiac disease may be characterized by acute, severe episodes of profuse, watery diarrhea and vomiting. This situation is referred to as a _____.

57. Identify the goals of therapy in short bowel syndrome.

a.

b.

c.

IV. Application, Analysis, and Synthesis of Essential Concepts

A. Clinical Situation: Manuel, age 3 years, is brought to the well-child clinic with the complaint of constipation.

1. To help confirm the medical diagnosis of constipation, you would begin your nursing assessment with questions regarding which factors?

a.

b.

c.

d.

B. Clinical Situation: Shane, age 11 months, is admitted to the pediatric unit for treatment of Hirschsprung disease.

1. What are the nursing goals in caring for Shane?

a.

b.

c.

d.

2. When preparing the parents for the medical treatment Shane will receive for his disease, the nurse would intervene by teaching that the repair of this defect is done in three stages. What are they?

a.

b.

c.

C. Clinical Situation: Stefanie, age 2 months, is admitted for treatment of gastroesophageal reflux (GER).

1. Positioning is the recommended method of managing GER. You would intervene by teaching Stefanie's parents about positioning. What would you teach them?

2. The nursing goals for Stefanie are:

a.

b.

c.

d.

D. Clinical Situation: Gerard, age 5 years, was admitted for treatment of appendicitis.

1. When assessing Gerard's pain, the nurse knows that the most reliable estimate of pain is the _____.

2. How will the nurse assess when to request discontinuance of Gerard's intermittent gastric decompression?

   a.

   b.

E. Experiential Exercise: Spend a day in an ambulatory pediatric clinic. To direct your nursing activities more constructively, differentiate between the two chronic intestinal disorders, ulcerative colitis and Crohn disease, by completing the following chart.

	Ulcerative Colitis	Crohn's Disease
Pathologic changes	1.	2.
Rectal bleeding	3.	4.
Diarrhea	5.	6.
Pain	7.	8.
Anorexia	9.	10.
Weight loss	11.	12.
Growth retardation	13.	14.

F. Clinical Situation: Samuel, age 11 years, is admitted to the pediatric unit with a diagnosis of hepatitis B.
   1. Nursing goals for Samuel's care depend on what three factors?

      a.

      b.

      c.

2. The emphasis of nursing care is on encouraging:

G. Experiential Exercise: Care for a child with a cleft lip or palate.
   1. Why does feeding pose a special challenge to the nurse?

   2. Identify the nursing goals in the postoperative period.

      a.

      b.

      c.

      d.

   3. What evaluation data would give evidence of achievement of the goal "Prevent trauma to suture line"?

H. Experiential Exercise: Care for a child who has hypertrophic pyloric stenosis.
   1. What nursing interventions do you use to achieve the nursing goal of preventing vomiting?

      a.

      b.

      c.

      d.

   2. What is the rationale for placing the patient in a head-elevated position after feeding?

   3. What nursing diagnosis reflects the effects of hospitalization on the patient?

   4. The patient is going home tomorrow, and the parents have been taught the home care of the child. How would you evaluate whether your interventions were effective in teaching the parents home care?

I. Clinical Situation: Jason, age 8 months, is admitted to the emergency room with signs of intermittent abdominal pain, vomiting, and currant-jelly stools. A diagnosis of intussusception is made.

1. As soon as the diagnosis of intussusception is made, the nurse begins to prepare Jason's parents for his immediate hospitalization, the barium enema, and the possibility of surgery. What specific nursing interventions would adequately prepare the parents to deal with each of these stressors?

    a. Hospitalization—

    b. Barium enema—

J. Clinical Situation: Patricia, age 3 years, is admitted with a diagnosis of celiac disease.

1. Patricia is going to have a peroral jejunal biopsy to definitely determine diagnosis. The nurse would intervene by preparing Patricia for this exam by:

    a.

    b.

    c.

2. A gluten-free diet usually produces dramatic clinical improvement within 2 weeks. Your nursing goal is to teach Patricia and her parents to adhere to this diet. What foods must she avoid?

V. Suggested Readings

Anson O, and others: Celiac disease: parental knowledge and attitudes of dietary compliance, Pediatrics 85(1):98-103, 1990.

> Forty-three parents of children with celiac disease were interviewed in this study to ascertain their knowledge, attitudes, and dietary behavior. Parents of compliant patients were compared with those of noncompliant patients. As a result, suggestions for increasing dietary compliance in celiac patients were presented.

Orenstein SR: Effects on behavior state of prone versus seated positioning for infants with gastroesophageal reflux, Pediatrics 85(5):765-767, 1990.

> Forty-eight infants younger than 6 months of age with reflux were included in this study. To compare the therapeutic effects of positioning on reflux, 24 infants were continuously positioned in the prone position and 24 infants were continuously positioned in the seated position during a 120-minute monitored postprandial period. The study showed that the prone infants had a significantly increased amount of sleep time and a significantly decreased amount of crying time.

Orenstein SR: Prone positioning in infant gastroesophageal reflux: is elevation of the head worth the trouble? Pediatr 117(2):184-187, 1990.

> One hundred babies less than 6 months of age who were being examined for reflux with an intraluminal esophageal pH probe while the babies were in each of the two positions (flat-prone, head-elevated prone) were included in the study. The babies were examined during a 2-hour postprandial period and a fasting period. There were no significant differences between the flat prone and the head-elevated prone position for any of the pH probe measurements.

Chapter 24

The Child with Cardiovascular Dysfunction

I. Chapter Overview

Chapter 24 introduces nursing considerations essential to the care of the child experiencing cardiovascular dysfunction. This is important, because it is estimated that congenital heart disease occurs in 8 to 10 of every thousand live births, and the acquired conditions affect children of virtually every age group. At the completion of this chapter, the student should have a knowledge of the structural and physiologic changes associated with the various cardiac disorders and will be able to develop appropriate nursing interventions for a child with cardiovascular dysfunction.

II. Learning Objectives

Upon completion of this chapter, it is expected that the student will be able to:

1. Design a plan for assisting a child during a cardiac diagnostic procedure.

2. Demonstrate an understanding of the hemodynamics, distinctive manifestations, and therapeutic management of congenital heart disease.

3. Outline a plan of care for an infant or child with congestive heart failure.

4. Describe the care for an infant or a child with a congenital heart defect.

5. Describe the care for a child who has hypoxia.

6. Discuss the role of the nurse in helping the child and family cope with congenital heart disease.

7. Discuss the assessment and management of hypertension in children and adolescents.

8. Contrast the causes and mechanisms of shock in children.

9. Outline a plan of care for the child with Kawasaki disease.

III. Review of Essential Concepts

1. A complication that the nurse might assess following a cardiac catheterization is:
    a. cardiac dysrhythmia
    b. rapidly rising blood pressure
    c. hypostatic pneumonia
    d. congestive heart failure

2. The two structures that influence the flow of blood in fetal circulation are the _____ _____ and the _____.

3. ___ In fetal circulation, the pressure on the left side of the heart exceeds the pressure on the right side. (true or false)

4. The congenital heart defects are divided into types based on the alterations in circulation. They are _____ and _____.

5. An acyanotic heart defect is one in which there is a _____ to _____ shunting of the blood.

6. A cyanotic heart defect is one in which there is a _____ to _____ shunting of the blood.

7. Match the following physical consequences of congenital heart disease with the underlying etiologies. (Answers may be used more than once; more than one answer may apply.)
   a. ___ growth retardation
   b. ___ recurrent respiratory infection
   c. ___ exercise intolerance
   d. ___ dyspnea
   e. ___ cyanosis
   f. ___ tachypnea
   g. ___ feeding problems
   h. ___ clubbing
   i. ___ tachycardia
   j. ___ polycythemia
      1) inadequate nutrient intake and increased caloric requirements
      2) pulmonary vascular congestion
      3) increased pulmonary resistance
      4) compensatory mechanism to increase oxygenation
      5) deoxygenation of blood
      6) compensatory mechanism to increase cardiac output
      7) chronic hypoxia

8. The six most common acyanotic congenital heart defects are:

9. Congestive heart failure is defined as:

10. The most common cause of congestive heart failure in children is _____ _____ secondary to structural abnormalities.

11. The two classifications of congestive heart failure are:
    a.

    b.

12. Related to impaired myocardial functioning, one of the earliest signs of decompensation to assess is _____.

13. Cardiac failure may lead to pulmonary congestion, producing such signs as:

14. Systemic congestion is a primary consequence of right-sided failure and is reflected in _____ and _____.

15. List the four goals of the therapeutic management of congestive heart failure.
    a.

    b.

    c.

    d.

16. What four interventions would the nurse use to help the parents and child adjust to the diagnosis of congenital heart disease?
    a.

    b.

    c.

    d.

17. The most common causative agent of bacterial endocarditis is _____.

18. The major sequela to rheumatic fever is heart damage, especially scarring of the _____.

19. Prevention or treatment of _____ _____infection prevents rheumatic fever.

20. Diagnosis of rheumatic fever is based on the presence of two major manifestations or one major and two minor manifestations as identified by the _____ criteria, in combinations with evidence of a recent _____ infection. The most objective evidence supporting a recent streptococcal infection is an elevated or rising _____ titer.

21. Define the following terms:
    a. Low-density lipoproteins (LDLs)

    b. High-density lipoproteins (HDLs)

22. The three classifications of cardiac dysrhythmias are:
    a.

    b.

    c.

23. Identify the initial nursing responsibility in relation to the cardiac dysrhythmias.

24. The diagnosis of hypertension in children and adolescents primarily involves the assessment of the _____ during every physical examination.

25. _____ to correct the underlying defect is the most common treatment for secondary hypertension. Essential or primary hypertension is commonly treated by _____ therapy.

26. Mucocutaneous lymph node syndrome, also known as _____, primarily affects the _____ system.

27. There is no specific diagnostic laboratory test for Kawasaki disease, so the diagnosis is based on the presence of five or six characteristic symptoms, which must always include an elevated _____.

28. In the acute stage and the recovery period of Kawasaki disease, nursing interventions include the administration of large doses of _____ and _____.

29. The physiologic consequences of shock are:
a.

b.

c.

30. The three stages or phases of shock are:
a.

b.

c.

31. ___ The most common type of shock in children is cardiogenic shock. (true or false)

32. Identify the three major goals of therapeutic management of shock.
a.

b.

c.

33. Anaphylaxis results from _____ _____ _____.

34. Identify early cutaneous signs of anaphylaxis.

35. ___ A criterion used to establish the diagnosis of toxic shock syndrome is a diffuse macular rash. (true or false)

36. The clinical manifestations of Henoch-Schonlein purpura are grouped into four categories. Name them.
a.

b.

c.

d.

IV. Application, Analysis, and Synthesis of Essential Concepts

A. Clinical Situation: Carolyn, 7 years old, is admitted to the pediatric unit for a cardiac catheterization on the following morning. She is accompanied by her parents. Both Carolyn and her parents appear anxious. A basic nursing assessment is performed.

1. In addition to the basic data, what three factors need to be assessed before giving Carolyn procedural information?
a.

b.

c.

2. Carolyn undergoes her cardiac catheterization and returns to the pediatric unit at noon. She appears drowsy and has a pressure dressing on her right groin area. The most important nursing responsibility associated with the postprocedural care of Carolyn would be the detection of complications. Identify the rationale(s) for each of the following nursing interventions or observations.
a. Frequent vital signs—

b. Monitor blood pressure, especially for hypotension—

c. Assess pulses distal to the catheterization site—

d. Assess the temperature and color of affected extremity—

B. Experiential Exercise: Spend a day in an outpatient cardiac clinic to observe the role of the nurse in the management of children with cardiac dysfunction.
1. Place C before the following clinical manifestations that might indicate the presence of a congenital heart defect in an infant or young child.
Mark X before incorrect answers.
   a. ___ growth retardation
   b. ___ bradycardia
   c. ___ difficulty with feeding
   d. ___ dyspnea
   e. ___ weak cry
   f. ___ bradypnea
   g. ___ decreased exercise tolerance
   h. ___ cyanosis
   i. ___ dry, hot skin
   j. ___ frequent respiratory infections
2. Identify the factors in a child's history that might be associated with an abnormally high incidence of congenital heart disease.
   a. Prenatal factors—

   b. Genetic factors—

3. What clinical manifestations might be seen in a child who is brought to the clinic with a diagnosed ventricular septal defect?

C. Experiential Exercise: Care for a hospitalized child with congestive heart failure.
1. Why would a child with congestive heart failure be placed on a regimen of oral digitalis and diuretics?

a. Digitalis—

b. Diuretics—

2. Since the margin of safety between the therapeutic and toxic dose of digitalis is narrow, the primary goal of the nurse is to prevent digitalis intoxication. What four nursing interventions would accomplish this goal?
   a.

   b.

   c.

   d.

3. What is the primary rationale for the nurse monitoring potassium levels in patients receiving potassium-losing diuretics and digoxin?

4. What signs would the nurse assess to detect digoxin toxicity in children?

5. For each of the following nursing goals, identify at least two appropriate nursing interventions that would be used when caring for a child with congestive heart failure.
   a. Assist in measures to improve cardiac functioning—

   b. Decrease cardiac demands—

c. Improve ventilation and oxygen supply–

d. Eliminate excess fluid and prevent fluid accumulation–

D. Clinical Situation: Julie, an 8-year-old black child, was admitted to the pediatric unit 5 days ago because of fatigue, low-grade fever, and joint pain. A heart murmur and subcutaneous nodules were discovered during her admission assessment. Laboratory tests, including an ESR, C-reactive protein, and ASO titer, helped confirm the diagnosis of rheumatic fever.
   1. The nurse is developing a home-care plan for Julie that includes the interventions listed below. Match each intervention to its appropriate rationale. (Answers may be used more than once; more than one answer may apply.)
   Rationale
   a. _____ prevention of permanent cardiac damage
   b. _____ prevention of recurrences of the disease
   c. _____ eradication of hemolytic streptococci
   d. _____ palliation of symptoms
   e. _____ provision of emotional support
      Interventions
      1) Administer antibiotics as ordered.
      2) Administer salicylates as needed.
      3) Enforce bed rest in the acute phase.
      4) Initiate prophylactic measures before dental work.
      5) Use a bed cradle.
      6) Prepare child for periodic multiple injections.
      7) Position child with pillows.
      8) Explain the temporary nature of all symptoms except cardiac involvement.
      9) Schedule activities to provide for adequate rest.
E. Clinical Situation: Johnny, age 3 years, is admitted to the pediatric unit with a diagnosis of Kawasaki disease. Upon admission, it is noted that Johnny has a fever of 102.5° F, a diffuse rash particularly evident on his trunk, and an enlargement of the cervical lymph nodes.

1. The six criteria used in establishing a diagnosis of Kawasaki disease are listed below. Develop a nursing diagnosis for each of these criteria.
   a. Fever for 5 or more days–

   b. Bilateral congestion of the ocular conjunctive without exudation–

   c. Changes of the mucous membranes of the oral cavity, such as erythema, dryness, and fissuring of the lips; oropharyngeal reddening, or "strawberry tongue"–

   d. Changes in extremities, such as peripheral edema, peripheral erythema, desquamation of palms and soles, particularly periungual peeling–

   e. Polymorphous rash, primarily of the trunk–

   f. Cervical lymphadenopathy–

2. For each of the following nursing goals, identify at least four appropriate nursing interventions to be used when caring for Johnny.
   a. Control fever–

   b. Prevent dehydration–

   c. Minimize possible cardiac complications–

V. Suggested Readings

Mistretta EF, Stroud S: Hypercholesterolemia in children: risk and management, Pediatr Nurs 16(2):152-154, 1990.

> Hypercholesterolemia in children is currently a controversial issue because of the lack of longitudinal data to support long-term intervention. The authors review the available literature and discuss which children are at risk, along with options for their management.

Zalzstein E, and others: Once-daily versus twice-daily dosing of digoxin in the pediatric group, Pediatr 116(1):137-139, 1990.

> Serum concentrations and clinical observations in infants and children (aged 2 months to 5.3 years) during once-daily and twice-daily administration of digoxin were compared in this study. The authors found no significant difference between a once-daily and a twice-daily maintenance dose of digoxin.

Zeigler V: Adenosine in the pediatric population: nursing implications, Pediatr Nurs 17(6):600-602, 1991.

> The author reviews the pharmacology, diagnostic and therapeutic uses, and nursing implications of the new drug adenosine. Graphic illustrations of the effect of adenosine on tachydysrhythmias are included.

Chapter 25

The Child with Hematologic or Immunologic Dysfunction

I. Chapter Overview

Chapter 25 introduces nursing considerations essential to the care of the child experiencing a dysfunction of the blood or blood-forming organs. Since many of these conditions are inherited and chronic in nature, it is important for the student to understand the care of children with such disorders. The disorders discussed in this chapter often result in widespread systemic and structural responses within the body. A portion of the chapter deals with the hematologic system and its function, and provides an overview of the hematopoietic process and the function of the various blood cells. Upon completion of this chapter, the student will be able to formulate nursing goals and identify the responsibilities that would assist the child and his family in adjusting to a hematopoietic disorder and to prevent or cope with the resulting complications.

II. Learning Objectives

Upon completion of this chapter, it is expected that the student will be able to:

1. Distinguish between the various categories of anemia.

2. Describe the prevention of and care of the child with iron-deficiency anemia.

3. Compare the pathophysiology and care of children with sickle cell anemia and thalassemia major.

4. Describe the mechanisms of inheritance and nursing care of the child with hemophilia.

5. Relate the pathophysiology and clinical manifestations of leukemia.

6. Demonstrate an understanding of the rationale of therapies for neoplastic disease.

7. Outline a plan of care for the child with neoplastic disease and the family.

8. Contrast the pathophysiology and management of the immune-deficiency disorders.

9. List nursing precautions and responsibilities during blood transfusion.

10. Describe the types of bone marrow transplants.

III. Review of Essential Concepts

1. List the components of the complete blood count (CBC).
    a.

    b.

    c.

    d.

    e.

f.

g.

h.

i.

j.

k.

2. Anemia is defined as _____ volume or hemoglobin concentration to below normal levels.

3. Name the two basic categories of anemia and explain them.

   a.

   b.

4. List the basic causes or etiology of anemia.

   a.

   b.

   c.

5. To understand the discussion of anemia, the nurse must be familiar with the terminology. Match the following terms with their definitions by placing the appropriate number in the preceding blank.

   a. ___ normocytic
   b. ___ normochromic
   c. ___ microchromic
   d. ___ microcytic
   e. ___ hypochromic
   f. ___ hemolysis
   g. ___ intracorpuscular
   h. ___ extracorpuscular factor
   i. ___ macrocytic
   1) large size red blood cell (RBC)
   2) conditions outside RBC that cause hemolysis
   3) defect within RBC
   4) normal size RBC
   5) pale color RBC
   6) excessive destruction of RBC
   7) normal color RBC
   8) RBCs that are pale in color
   9) small size RBC

6. To assess and interpret laboratory studies for integration into her client assessment, the nurse must understand the following laboratory measures. Identify what is measured by each of these tests.

   a. Mean corpuscular volume (MCV)–

   b. Mean corpuscular hemoglobin (MCH)–

   c. Mean corpuscular hemoglobin concentration (MCHC)–

   d. Red blood cell (RBC)–

   e. Hemoglobin (HGB)–

   f. Hematocrit (Hct)–

   g. Reticulocyte count–

   h. White blood cell count (WBC)–

   i. Differential WBC count–

   j. Platelet count–

7. The basic physiologic defect caused by anemia is:

8. The clinical manifestations of anemia are directly attributable to tissue hypoxia. Identify these clinical manifestations.

   a. Four general symptoms

   b. Seven central-nervous-system manifestations

   c. Circulatory system manifestations

9. The four nursing goals for the care of the child with anemia are:

   a.

   b.

   c.

   d.

10. _____ is required for the production of hemoglobin.

11. Often a baby with iron deficiency anemia is called a "milk baby." What is the meaning of this term?

12. The side effects of oral iron therapy are:

13. The main nursing goal regarding diet is:

14. When the proper dose of supplemental iron is reached, the stools usually turn a _____ .

15. List and define the two most common forms of sickle cell disease.

    a.

    b.

16. The basic defect in sickle cell anemia is the red blood cell changes into a _____ red cell.

17. The sickling response is preventable under conditions of adequate _____ and _____ .

18. The basic pathologic changes from sickle cell anemia are primarily the result of:

    a.

    b.

19. Sickle cell crisis is usually precipitated by an _____ .

20. The four types of sickle cell crisis are:

    a.

    b.

    c.

    d.

21. Because early identification of sickle cell anemia is essential, the _____ test is used for screening and case-finding.

22. Can oxygen administration reverse sickling of red blood cells?

23. What is the possible negative effect of prolonged oxygen administration for the sickle cell patient?

24. Twenty to thirty percent of children with sickle cell disease under age 5 die mainly from _____ .

25. Thalassemias are classified according to the _____ that is affected. Thalassemia major or _____ is a severe anemia that is not _____ with life.

26. If you trace the pathologic process of thalassemia major, you will see the following sequence:

    a. There is defective hemoglobin A, synthesis of which disintegrates, causing damage to the _____ which causes severe _____ . To compensate for the hemolytic process, the bone marrow produces large numbers of immature red blood cells that have a severely shortened _____ . The increase of _____ , the iron-containing pigment from the breakdown of hemoglobin, results in an increased amount of iron in the blood. The body stores the iron (a process called _____), resulting in cellular damage.

27. _____ , an iron-chelating agent, is given to the child with thalassemia to obviate hemosiderosis.

28. The definition of hemophilia is:

29. The two most common forms of hemophilia are classic hemophilia and Christmas disease. _____ accounts for 75% of all cases of hemophilia. What factors are defective in each form?

    a. Classic hemophilia—

    b. Christmas disease—

30. Hemophilia is transmitted as an _____
_____.
The most common pattern of transmission
is between an unaffected male and a carrier
female.

31. The most frequent site of bleeding is the
_____; such a bleed is called
a _____.

32. One of the major causes of death in the
hemophiliac is _____.

33. The primary therapy for the hemophiliac is
preventing spontaneous bleeding by:

34. _____ is the drug of choice for the child
with hemophilia A.

35. Thrombocytopenic purpura is characterized
by:
a.

b.

36 ___ Disseminated intravascular coagulation
is a primary disease. (true or false)

37. The most important prognostic factors in
determining long-term survival for children
with ALL are:

38. The two basic pathologic factors that occur
in leukemia are:
a.

b.

39. The four main consequences of bone marrow
dysfunction are _____,
_____, _____
_____, and _____.

40. The clinical manifestations that result from
the bone marrow dysfunction are:

41. Invasion of the meninges results in
_____.

42. Definitive diagnosis of leukemia is based on
_____
or _____.

43. List the three phases of chemotherapeutic
therapy for leukemia.

44. The central nervous system preventive and
consolidation phase of therapy is directed
toward what anatomic area that is protected
from systemic chemotherapy?

45. What are the most common drugs and other
therapies used in each of the three phases of
chemotherapy?
a. Induction–

b. Sanctuary–

c. Maintenance–

46. Differentiate between Hodgkin disease and
non-Hodgkin lymphoma.

47. Hodgkin disease is characterized by painless _____.

48. The primary modalities of therapy for
Hodgkin disease are _____ and
_____ used alone or in combination.

49. The human immunodeficiency virus (HIV)
is transmitted through _____
with blood or blood products and _____
_____ in which blood and semen
mix, and through maternal _____
_____.

50. Seventy-seven percent of the cases of
acquired immune deficiency syndrome
(AIDS) in children are the result of
_____ transmission.

51. Nursing considerations are primarily directed at _____.

52. What is the etiology, therapeutic management, and prognosis of AIDS?

a. Etiology—

b. Therapeutic management—

c. Prognosis—

53. Severe combined immunodeficiency disease (SCID) is defined as:

54. The only definitive treatment of SCID is a
_____.

55. Wiskott-Aldrich syndrome is characterized by three abnormalities. List them.

a.

b.

c.

56. List the major categories of immediate reactions to a blood transfusion.

a.

b.

c.

d.

e.

f.

g.

57. Three types of bone marrow transplants are:

a.

b.

c.

IV. Application, Analysis, and Synthesis of Essential Concepts

A. Clinical Situation: Regina, age 4 years, is admitted to the pediatric unit for diagnosis and treatment of possible anemia.

1. Regina will be undergoing a battery of blood tests. The nursing goal of preparing the child for these tests can be accomplished by the following nursing interventions:

a.

b.

c.

2. What nursing diagnoses are appropriate for Regina?

a.

b.

B. Clinical Situation: Tonisha, age 3 years, is hospitalized with sickle cell anemia.

1. Since the major medical and nursing goals are to prevent deoxygenation and dehydration, what nursing interventions will you initiate to accomplish each of these goals?

a. Prevent tissue deoxygenation—

b. Prevent dehydration—

2. Tonisha has lapsed into sickle cell crisis. What nursing diagnoses are appropriate for Tonisha?

a.

b.

3. What would be the evaluative data to support achievement of the goal "minimize physical exertion"?

C. Clinical Situation: Ryan, age 3 years, is hospitalized for treatment of his hemophilia A.

1. In addition to observing for signs of hemarthrosis, the nurse should intervene in teaching the family the other signs of internal hemorrhage. What are these signs and symptoms?

2. What emergency measures (interventions) could the family institute for a bleeding episode in addition to factor replacement? Include a rationale for each one.

   a.

   b.

   c.

D. Clinical Situation: Billy, age 7 years, is hospitalized with a diagnosis of leukemia.
   1. List the nursing goals that are appropriate for the nursing diagnosis "High risk for injury related to interference with cell proliferation."

      a.

      b.

      c.

   2. What nursing interventions would be appropriate to achieve the goal of "maintaining skin integrity"?

      a.

      b.

      c.

E. Clinical Situation: Tony, age 4 months, is being treated for AIDS.
   1. One of the nursing goals for Tony is to educate the parents, the family, and the public regarding precautions to prevent transmission of the virus. List the precautions necessary when coming in contact with body fluids.

      a.

      b.

      c.

      d.

      e.

      f.

   2. List the nursing diagnoses for Tony and his family.

a.

b.

c.

d.

V. Suggested Readings

McConnell EA: Leukocyte studies: what the counts can tell you, Nursing 86 16(3):42-43, 1986.

> The article briefly reviews and explains the function of each of the five types of white cells. The white blood cell count and the differential count are explained, and their use in identifying the patient's diagnosis is explored.

Morrison RA: Update on sickle cell disease: incidence of addiction and choice of opioid in pain management, Pediatr Nurs 17(5):503, 1991.

> Two important concerns in pain management of children with sickle cell disease — addiction and choice of drug — are reviewed. The author bases her conclusions on 13 years of experience and more than 630 pediatric patients with pain caused by this disease. The author contends that addiction is not an increased problem in this population. The author also emphasizes contraindication of the use of meperidine with sickle cell clients.

Stiehm ER, and Vink P: Transmission of human immunodeficiency virus infection by breast-feeding, Pediatr 118(3):410-411, 1991.

> These authors present the first case in the United States of transmission of HIV by breast-feeding. They discuss implications for breast-feeding in high-risk mothers.

Wimberley TH, Parks BR: Iron preparations: it's elementary, my dear, Pediatr Nurs 17(3)274-275, 1991.

> The authors discuss iron requirements, types of preparations, dosage, and adverse effects of iron therapy. Iron-deficiency anemia has an excellent prognosis if identified early and if iron is supplied by the correct preparation and by the correct dosage.

Chapter 26

The Child with Genitourinary Dysfunction

I.   Chapter Overview

Chapter 26 introduces the nursing considerations essential to the care of the child who is experiencing renal dysfunction. Students need to understand these illnesses because diseases of the kidney are relatively common in children. Disturbances in renal function often are the most difficult to master because the complex anatomy and physiology of the kidney are essential to understanding how the pathologic process progresses. At the completion of this chapter the student will understand the tests used to assess renal function, the more common disorders of renal function, the various types of dialysis, and renal transplantation. The student will be able to care for the child who is experiencing renal dysfunction in the practicum setting.

II.   Learning Objectives

Upon completion of this chapter, it is expected that the student will be able to:

1.   Describe the various factors that contribute to urinary tract infections in infants and children.

2.   Demonstrate an understanding of the causes and mechanisms of edema formation in nephrotic syndrome.

3.   Outline a nursing care plan for a child with nephrotic syndrome.

4.   Compare child with minimal-change nephrotic syndrome with the child with acute glomeru-lonephritis in terms of clinical manifestations and nursing care.

5.   Contrast the causes, complications, and management of acute and chronic renal failure.

6.   Discuss the preoperative preparation of the child and parents when the child has a structural defect of the genitourinary tract.

7.   List the types of renal failure.

8.   Recognize signs of kidney transplant rejection.

III. Review of Essential Concepts

1.   The single most important host factor influencing the occurrence of a urinary tract infection is _____.

2.   ___ The presence of alkaline urine inhibits the growth of bacteria. (true or false)

3.   The four objectives of the therapeutic management of the child with a urinary tract infection are:
a.

b.

c.

d.

4.   Obstruction of the urinary system can be caused by:

a.

b.

c.

d.

5. Define hydronephrosis:

6. The massive edema seen in nephrotic syndrome is a result of:
   a. inability to excrete excess sodium
   b. hypoalbuminemia leading to decreases in osmotic pressure
   c. narrowing of the renal afferent arterioles
   d. decreased urine output leading to increased intravascular volume

7. A clinical manifestation of nephrotic syndrome is:
   a. hypertension
   b. coffee-colored urine
   c. proteinuria
   d. low specific gravity

8. _____ are the primary therapeutic agents used to treat nephrotic syndrome.

9. A common side effect of steroid therapy is:
   a. growth retardation
   b. hypotension
   c. renal calculi
   d. constipation

10. Match the clinical manifestation with the renal disease in which it is seen.
    a. ___ hypertension
    b. ___ hematuria
    c. ___ anasarca
    d. ___ azotemia
    e. ___ increased serum lipid levels
       1) nephrotic syndrome
       2) acute glomerulonephritis

11. List the methods used in the diagnostic evaluation of acute glomerulonephritis.
    a.

    b.

    c.

    d.

    e.

f.

g.

12. ___ Water intake is restricted in all children with acute glomerulonephritis. (true or false)

13. ___ Hypertension is a common result of glomerulonephritis. (true or false)

14. The function of the _____ is the reabsorption of substances, and the function of the _____ is filtration.

15. ___ Urinary tract infections are commonly seen in patients with obstructive uropathy. (true or false)

16. _____ represents one of the most frequent causes of acute renal failure in childhood.

17. The primary site of injury in hemolytic uremic syndrome is _____.

18. List the clinical manifestations of hemolytic uremic syndrome.
    a.

    b.

    c.

    d.

    e.

    f.

    g.

    h.

19. The anemia seen in hemolytic uremic syndrome results from:

20. A prerenal cause of acute renal failure is:
    a. renal hypoplasia
    b. Alport syndrome
    c. dehydration
    d. obstructive uropathy

21. The prime clinical manifestation of acute renal failure is _____.

22. ___ Metabolic alkalosis is commonly seen in patients with acute renal failure. (true or false)

23. Treatment of acute renal failure is directed toward:
    a.

b.

c.

24. Two major complications of acute renal failure are _____ and _____.

25. ___ Children with chronic renal failure are placed on high-protein, high-calorie diets. (true or false)

26. Dialysis is:

27. The types of dialysis are:
    a.

    b.

    c.

28. _____ is now an acceptable and effective means of therapy in the pediatric age group.

IV. Application, Analysis, and Synthesis of Essential Concepts

A. Clinical Situation: Barry, age 3 months, is brought to the pediatrician by his mother, who says that for the past few days Barry has been eating poorly, is running a high temperature, is sleeping much more than usual, and seems to be voiding large amounts. A urine culture is obtained. The pediatrician believes that Barry may have a urinary tract infection secondary to an obstruction and has him admitted to the hospital.

1. The nursing assessment yielded several signs and symptoms of renal disease in Barry. List them.
    a.

    b.

    c.

    d.

    e.

2. Why did the pediatrician suspect that Barry may have obstructive uropathy?

3. The most important nursing goal when caring for children with urinary tract infections is _____.

4. Formulate two nursing diagnoses for the child with a urinary tract infection.
    a.

    b.

5. List the nursing interventions used to care for Barry.
    a.

    b.

    c.

    d.

    e.

    f.

    g.

6. How would you evaluate whether the interventions were successful in teaching Barry's parents how to prevent recurrence?

B. Experiential Exercise: Care for a child who has minimal-change nephrotic syndrome.

1. Formulate one nursing diagnosis that is related to the presence of edema in this child.

2. List one nursing goal related to the susceptibility of this child to infection.

3. List the nursing interventions used to provide good nutrition to this patient.
    a.

    b.

    c.

    d.

    e.

    f.

4. What is the rationale for providing meticulous skin care?

5. List four nursing interventions aimed at conserving the child's energy.
   a.

   b.

   c.

   d.

6. What interventions should be developed to prepare the child for discharge?

7. How do you evaluate whether the interventions were successful in preparing the parents for discharge of the child?

C. Clinical Situation: Tina, age 6 years, was admitted to the pediatric unit. Tina's history reveals that she had a severe sore throat and had been receiving antibiotics. Her mother stopped giving them when Tina felt better. Her admitting diagnosis is acute glomerulonephritis. She is anuric and has severe hypertension. It is believed that she has acute renal failure, secondary to the nephritis.
1. What nursing intervention might have prevented the occurrence of acute glomerulonephritis in Tina?

2. Formulate one nursing goal related to the alteration of fluid balance in Tina.

3. List four nursing interventions to provide diversion in Tina.

a.

b.

c.

d.

4. List the nursing interventions necessary to maintain fluid balance in Tina while she has acute renal failure.
   a.

   b.

   c.

   d.

   e.

   f.

5. What is the rationale for placing Tina on a low-protein diet while she has acute renal failure?

6. How would you evaluate whether the nurse was successful at supporting the family?

D. Clinical Situation: Betsy is a patient on the pediatric unit. She was first admitted to the unit with hemolytic uremic syndrome. She has recovered from the primary disease but now appears to have chronic renal failure. She is to be taught how to perform home peritoneal dialysis.
1. What were the signs and symptoms of hemolytic uremic syndrome that Betsy probably exhibited?

2. Formulate one nursing diagnosis related to the susceptibility of Betsy to infection.

3. Identify two nursing goals for Betsy related to diet and elimination.

a.

b.

4. List the nursing interventions to be developed to promoted optimum home care for Betsy.

a.

b.

c.

d.

e.

f.

g.

5. List the nursing interventions aimed at treating Betsy's hypertension.

a.

b.

c.

d.

6. How would you evaluate whether nursing interventions were successful in assisting the child with the stresses of chronic renal failure?

a.

b.

c.

E. Clinical Situation: Richard Patucci, age 3 years, is admitted for treatment of a Wilm tumor.

1. Because surgery is performed within 24 to 48 hours after admission, the nurse must prepare Richard's parents for this procedure. List at least one nursing intervention to accomplish this.

2. Because Richard is prone to intestinal obstruction, what postoperative nursing interventions are appropriate?

a.

b.

c.

V. Suggested Readings

Horton H, and others: Hypospadias: when baby boys need surgery, RN 90(6):48-51, 1990.

> Nursing goals and responsibilities in the care of infant boys after surgery for hypospadias is the focus of this article. Immediate postoperative nursing care through home care is discussed.

Suddaby EC, and others: Continuous hemofiltration in infants and children, Pediatr Nurs 16(1):79-82, 1990.

> The technique of continuous arteriovenous hemofiltration (CAVH) in the treatment of acute renal failure is explored in this article. Explanation of the CAVH system and its use in the pediatric population is included. A detailed guide for nursing care of the child and his family is discussed.

Chapter 27

The Child with Cerebral Dysfunction

I. Chapter Overview

Chapter 27 introduces nursing considerations essential to the care of the child experiencing cerebral dysfunction. Since the brain is the center for multiple vital body functions, any disturbance in this regulating, controlling, and communicating mechanism can produce alterations in the way in which the system receives, integrates, and responds to stimuli entering the system. Since an alteration in the level of consciousness is a common finding in many cerebral disturbances, the student will be introduced to methods used to assess and diagnose neurologic function. At the completion of this chapter the student will be able to develop nursing goals and responsibilities that help the child and his family to effectively cope with the stressors imposed by an alteration in cerebral function.

II. Learning Objectives

Upon completion of this chapter, it is expected that the student will be able to:

1. Describe the various modalities for assessment of cerebral function.

2. Differentiate between the stages of consciousness.

3. Formulate a plan of care for the unconscious child.

4. Distinguish between the types of head injuries and the serious complications.

5. Describe the nursing care of a child with a tumor of the central nervous system.

6. Outline a plan of care for the child with bacterial meningitis.

7. Differentiate between the various types of seizure disorders.

8. Demonstrate an understanding of the manifestations of a convulsive disorder and the management of a child with such a disorder.

9. Describe preoperative and postoperative care of a child with hydrocephalus.

III. Review of Essential Concepts

1. List the aspects of assessment for cerebral dysfunction.
   a.

   b.

   c.

2. The early signs and symptoms of increased intracranial pressure are subtle and assume many patterns. List these signs and symptoms for the younger and older child.
   a. Younger child—

b. Older child–

3. As intracranial pressure becomes progressively worse, what signs would you expect to assess?

4. Because it is difficult to assess cerebral function in the infant and small child, what methods are employed?
a.

b.

c.

d.

5. The _____ and _____ will contribute to the assessment of cerebral function.

6. Older children can be evaluated by the usual methods of neurologic examination, including _____ _____.

7. List and define the two components of consciousness and explain them.
a.

b.

8. Level of consciousness (LOC) is determined primarily by:

9. List the terms that describe LOC.

10. The Glasgow coma scale (GCS) consists of what three areas of assessment?
a.

b.

c.

11. The purpose of the neurologic examination is to:

12. What areas are assessed in performing a neurologic examination?

13. The sudden appearance of a fixed and dilated pupil is a _____.

14. List the diagnostic procedures, other than blood tests, that are used to assess cerebral function.
a.

b.

c.

d.

e.

f.

g.

h.

i.

j.

k.

l.

m.

15. One of the primary concerns when caring for an unconscious patient is to maintain a _____.

16. List and define the types of head injuries.
   a.

   b.

   c.

17. List the major complications of trauma to the head.
   a.

   b.

   c.

   d.

18. Vascular rupture may occur even in minor head injuries, causing hemorrhage between the skull and cerebral surfaces. Why is the accumulation of blood between the skull and cerebral surfaces dangerous?

19. What are the clinical manifestations of epidural hemorrhage in children?

20. The accumulate blood is called a _____.

21. A subdural hemorrhage is bleeding _____, usually as a result of rupture of the _____.

22. Another major complication of head trauma is _____.

23. If cerebral edema is not detected and relieved, what is the consequence to the brain tissue?

24. What diagnostic test is essential in diagnosing neurologic trauma?

25. The most important nursing consideration in caring for a child with a head injury is _____.

26. The major pulmonary changes that occur in drowning are directly related to:

27. The major problems caused by near-drowning are:
   a.

   b.

   c.

28. Most drownings of children can be _____ with adequate supervision.

29. The major infratentorial tumors of childhood are:

30. Because the signs and symptoms of brain tumors are related to increasing intracranial pressure, infants with brain tumors do not display easily detectable symptoms. Why not?

31. The most diagnostic procedure for a brain tumor is the _____.

32. The treatment of choice for brain tumors is total _____.

33. When the temperature is elevated in a patient after removal of a brain tumor, the nurse would suspect an _____.

34. Headache may be severe after surgery in the patient with brain tumor. The headaches are largely caused by _____.

35. Why is the Trendelenburg position contraindicated in the patient who has had a brain tumor removed?

36. The primary site for a neuroblastoma is within the _____ or _____.

37. Diagnostic evaluation of neuroblastoma is aimed at locating the _____ and _____.

38. Neuroblastomas often excrete catecholamines. How is the presence of catecholamines detected?

39. Identify the three methods employed to treat neuroblastoma.
    a.

    b.

    c.

40. Because of the frequency of _____ _____, prognosis for neuroblastoma is poor.

41. What organisms are responsible for 95% of the cases of bacterial meningitis in children older than 2 months?
    a.

    b.

    c.

42. What form of meningitis is readily transmitted to others and by what vehicle?

43. A definitive diagnosis of meningococcal meningitis is made only by?

44. Identify the following statements regarding bacterial meningitis as true (T) or false (F).
    a. ___ Isolation is not needed for bacterial meningitis.
    b. ___ Seizures do not occur in affected children.
    c. ___ There are no vaccines for bacterial meningitis.

45. The treatment of aseptic meningitis is primarily _____.

46. Encephalitis can occur as a result of:
    a.

    b.

47. Reye syndrome usually follows a common viral illness such as _____ or _____.

48. Research has confirmed an association between the use of _____ and the incidence of Reye syndrome.

49. What are the dominant clinical manifestations of human immunodeficiency virus encephalopathy?

50. What are the two types of immunizing products available for rabies in humans?
    a.

    b.

51. The basic mechanism of seizures is that electric discharges caused by spontaneous electric discharge:

52. What are the two major categories of seizures?

53. Psychomotor seizures are characterized by:

54. The _____ is the most useful diagnostic tool for evaluating seizure disorders.

55. What are the goals of therapeutic management?
    a.

    b.

    c.

56. What is the action of anticonvulsive drugs?

57. What precautions should be taken if the anticonvulsive drug is discontinued?

58. How is the dosage of anticonvulsant drugs monitored?

59. The tonic-clonic seizure is also known as _____.

60. The generalized seizure that is characterized by a brief loss of consciousness with minimal or no alteration in muscle tone and that may go unrecognized is called _____ or _____.

61. Status epilepticus is defined as:

62. Seizure precautions include:

63. Define febrile seizures:

64. The majority of infants with craniosynostosis have _____ brain development.

65. _____ is a condition caused by an imbalance in the production and absorption of cerebrospinal fluid in the ventricular system, usually under increased pressure.

66. Although the causes of hydrocephalus are varied, the result is either:
    a.

    b.

67. The most commonly observed clinical manifestations of hydrocephalus in the infant include:
    a.

    b.

    c.

    d.

    e.

    f.

    g.

    h.

    i.

68. ____ The signs and symptoms of hydrocephalus in early and late childhood are caused by increased intracranial pressure. (true or false)

69. The primary diagnostic tools for detecting hydrocephalus are _____ and _____.

IV. Application, Analysis, and Synthesis of Essential Concepts

A. Clinical Situation: Beatrice McKinney, age 7 years, was admitted to the pediatric unit after sustaining head trauma in an automobile accident. When admitted, she was conscious and complaining that her head hurt.
1. Beatrice has begun to complain of a headache and nausea, blurred vision, and she seems drowsy. What nursing diagnosis would you formulate from this assessment data?

2. Beatrice is becoming increasingly confused, disoriented, and agitated. She is suddenly fearful of the monitoring machines at her bedside because she thinks they are "wild animals." Based on this assessment, what level of consciousness would best describe Beatrice?

B. Clinical Situation: Greta Kneisl, age 8 years, has been unconscious for 3 days as a result of head trauma.
1. List at least three nursing goals for the care of Greta.
    a.

    b.

    c.

    d.

    e.

    f.

    g.

h.

i.

j.

k.

l.

m.

n.

o.

p.

q.

r.

s.

t.

2. What parameters are assessed to monitor Greta's neurologic status?

3. What nursing interventions would achieve the nursing goal of "preventing" intracranial pressure"?
    a.

    b.

    c.

    d.

    e.

4. What is the rationale for placing the child on a water-filled mattress?

C. Experiential Exercise: Spend a day in an emergency room for pediatric clients. Answer the following questions and include specifics (examples, responses) to illustrate these concepts.
    1. Robin, age 3 years, sustained head trauma in a fall down some stairs. She is diagnosed as having a subdural hematoma and admitted to the pediatric unit.

a. Three important nursing observations are frequent examination of:

2. Tory, age 3 years, comes to the emergency room after being rescued from a swimming pool. After immediate resuscitation of the child to restore oxygen delivery to the cells, the nurse must be concerned about Tory's parents. What nursing interventions would help comfort the parents?

D. Clinical Situation: Eden Capwell, age 10 months, is admitted to the pediatric unit with a diagnosis of meningococcal meningitis.
    1. What clinical manifestations would you expect to assess in Eden?

2. Identify the major goals of therapeutic management to be used when caring for Eden.
    a.

    b.

    c.

    d.

    e.

    f.

    g.

    h.

    i.

    j.

E. Clinical Situation: Anita Sanchez, age 4 years, was admitted to the pediatric unit for diagnosis and treatment of a seizure disorder.
    1. To assist with Anita's diagnosis, the nurse should gather through a nursing history or through direct assessment what data?
        a.

b.

c.

d.

e.

f.

g.

2. While you are giving Anita a bath in bed, she begins to have a seizure. How would you intervene to care for Anita and prevent any injury to her?
   a.

   b.

   c.

   d.

   e.

   f.

3. Anita was diagnosed as having grand mal seizures and is placed on dilantin. The nurse would formulate a teaching plan regarding drug therapy. You would intervene by teaching the following points:
   a.

   b.

   c.

   d.

   e.

   f.

   g.

F. Clinical Situation: Adam Morrissey, a newborn, is transferred to the pediatric unit for hydrocephalus.
   1. Postoperative nursing interventions for the child with hydrocephalus include:
      a.

      b.

c.

d.

2. List the nursing diagnoses for Adam:
   a.

   b.

   c.

3. What evaluative data would reveal that the goal of "support the family" has been achieved?

V. Suggested Readings

Hinkle JL: Treating traumatic coma, Am J Nurs 86:551-556, 1986.

The most important function of the nurse and emergency medical personnel is to prevent ischemia of the brain after a traumatic head injury. The author presents the priorities of care to accomplish this goal. The methods of monitoring and lowering intracranial pressure are outlined. The nursing role in reducing intracranial pressure and in constant assessment of the cerebral status of the child is explored.

Scheinblum ST, Hammond M: The treatment of children with shunt infections: extraventricular drainage system care, Pediatr Nurs 16(2):139-143, 1990.

The authors review the use of internal shunt placement over several decades, then go on to focus on the problem of shunt infections. They thoroughly explore the treatment of these infections by using an extraventricular drainage system (EVD). The authors present nursing care considerations, especially the emotional concerns of the child and his family.

Shinaberger CS, and others: Young children who drown in hot tubs, spas, and whirlpools in California: a 26-year survey, Am J Pub Health 80(5):613-614, 1990.

Data for this survey were collected from 1960 to 1985 in Southern California. The survey identified 74 drowning victims during this period. The results of this survey indicate that residential hot tubs, spas, and whirlpools represent poorly recognized but high-risk drowning sites for young children. The authors suggest several preventive strategies.

Wintemute GJ, Wright MA: Swimming pool owners' opinion of strategies for prevention of drowning, Pediatrics 85(1):63-69, 1990.

Although mandatory cardiopulmonary resuscitation and placement of a barrier around pools are the two commonly suggested strategies for prevention of drowning, the authors of this study sought to assess what pool owners thought were appropriate strategies. A survey of 796 pool owners in Sacramento County found that a large majority of the owners favored mandatory CPR, but a small minority favored a mandatory barrier. The results yielded suggestions for specific directions for programs aimed at preventing swimming pool drownings.

Chapter 28

The Child with Endocrine Dysfunction

I. Chapter Overview

Chapter 28 introduces nursing considerations essential to the care of the child experiencing endocrine dysfunction. Since the hormones synthesized by this system affect numerous body organs, it is important for the student to gain an understanding of the care of children with this type of alteration in health. The conditions discussed in this chapter interfere with the body's ability to produce or respond to the major hormones. The discussion of pancreatic hormone secretion is limited to diabetes mellitus, a relatively common health problem of childhood. At the completion of this chapter, the student will be able to develop nursing goals and responsibilities that will help the child and his family develop effective coping responses to deal with these complex disorders.

II. Learning Objectives

Upon completion of this chapter, it is expected that the student will be able to:

1. Differentiate between the disorders caused by hypopituitary and hyperpituitary dysfunction.

2. Describe the manifestations of thyroid hypofunction and hyperfunction and the management of children with the disorders.

3. Distinguish between the manifestations of adrenal hypofunction and hyperfunction.

4. Differentiate among the various categories of diabetes mellitus.

5. Discuss the management and nursing care of the child with diabetes mellitus in the acute care setting.

6. Distinguish between hypoglycemia and a hyperglycemic reaction.

7. Design a teaching plan for a child with diabetes mellitus.

8. Formulate a teaching plan for instructing parents of a child with diabetes mellitus.

III. Review of Essential Concepts

1. The pituitary gland is also known as the _____ or _____ .

2. _____ is the most common cause of pituitary hyposecretion.

3. The main presenting complaint of hypopituitarism is _____ .

4. Diagnosis of hypopituitarism is based on absent or subnormal reserves of _____ _____ .

5. The therapeutic management of hypopituitarism is:

    a.

    b.

. Excess growth hormone before closure of epiphyseal shafts results in proportional _____; after closure of epiphyseal shafts results in _____, termed _____.

7. Children with a pituitary secreting tumor may also demonstrate signs of _____ _____.

8. The primary nursing responsibility regarding hypopituitarism and hyperpituitarism is:

9. The principal disorder of the posterior pituitary hypofunction is _____, which causes hyposecretion of antidiuretic hormone (ADH), producing a state of uncontrolled _____.

10. The cardinal signs of diabetes insipidus are _____ and _____.

11. The usual treatment of diabetes insipidus is hormone replacement with _____.

12. SIADH = _____, which results in_____and _____.

13. The _____ gland is the only endocrine gland capable of storing excess amounts of hormones for release as needed.

14. The main physiologic action of the thyroid hormone is _____ and thereby controls multiple processes of growth and tissue differentiation.

15. A goiter is:

The synthesis of thyroid hormone depends upon the availability of _____.

16. Graves disease is usually associated with an enlarged _____.

17. List the symptoms that may occur if the patient with thyroid hyperfunction develops thyrotoxicosis.

18. A possible complication of thyroidectomy is _____.

19. The objective of therapeutic management of hypoparathyroidism is to maintain normal serum _____ and _____ levels with minimum complications.

20. _____ can be secondary to chronic renal disease and congenital anomalies of the urinary tract.

21. Identify whether the following hormones are secreted by the adrenal medulla or the adrenal cortex by matching the following:
a. ___ glucocorticoids (cortisol)
b. ___ catecholamine (epinephrine)
c. ___ catecholamine (norepinephrine)
d. ___ mineralocorticoid (aldosterone)
e. ___ sex steroids
1) adrenal cortex
2) adrenal medulla

22. Identify whether the following clinical manifestations are indicative of (1) adrenocortical insufficiency or (2) hyperfunction of the adrenal gland.
a. ____ Increased irritability, headache, diffuse abdominal pain, weakness, nausea and vomiting, diarrhea, fever, and CNS symptoms
b. ___ Moon face; hyperglycemia; decreased protein stores, increased mobilization and use of fatty acids for energy; increased storage of adipose tissue; decreased inflammatory and allergic actions; regulation of fluid and electrolytes by promoting sodium retention and potassium excretion; increased gastric acid and pepsin; and suppression of lymphocytes, eosinophils, and basophils but increased neutrophils, erythrocytes, and thrombocytes

23. The administration of excessive amounts of exogenous corticosteroids can result in _____.

24. A characteristic sign of excess cortisol, whether from exogenous steroid therapy or malfunction of the adrenal gland, is the _____ face.

25. Untreated congenital adrenogenital hyperplasia results in early _____ maturation.

26. A sex is assigned to the child with adrenogenital hyperplasia that is consistent with the _____.

27. Urinary levels of 17-ketosteroids are abnormal in _____.

28. Pheochromocytomas arise from chromaffin cells of the adrenal medulla and there is a _____ transmission as an autosomal _____ trait.

29. The clinical manifestations of pheochromocytoma are caused by _____ _____.

30. The islets of Langerhans of the pancreas have three major functioning cells. List the hormone produced by each of these cells and its function.

a.

b.

c.

31. The three types of diabetes mellitus are:
   a.

   b.

   c.

32. Compare the characteristics of Type I and Type II diabetes mellitus by completing the following chart:

Characteristic	Type I (IDDM)	Type II (NIDDM)
Age of onset	a.	b.
Present in both parents	c.	d.
Presenting symptoms	e.	f.
Ketoacidosis	g.	h.

33. Trace the pathophysiology of diabetes mellitus by describing the etiology underlying each of the following physical consequences of the absence of insulin.
   a. Insulin is absent–

   b. Hyperglycemia–

   c. Glycosuria–

d. Polyuria–

e. Polydipsia–

f. Metabolizes proteins and fats–

g. Glycogenesis–

h. Polyphagia–

i. Ketonuria and acetone breath–

j. Metabolic acidosis–

34. What are the long-term complications of diabetes mellitus?
   a.
      1)

      2)

      3)

35. What are the three "polys" of diabetes mellitus?

36. Tests used to determine glycosuria are the _____ or _____.

37. ___ Postprandial blood glucose test is essential to establish a diagnosis of diabetes. (true or false)

38. _____ are designed to deliver fixed amounts of regular insulin continuously, thereby imitating the release of the hormone by the islet cells.

39. _____ (HBGM) has improved diabetes management and can be used successfully by children.

40. Exercise is beneficial to the diabetic child because it _____ blood sugar levels.

41. _____ is prescribed for home treatment of hypoglycemia.

42. Describe the Somogyi effect.

43. The therapeutic management of ketoacidosis consists of:
a.

b.

c.

d.

44. After hydrating the child, a normal serum _____ level must be reestablished.

45. Differentiate between ketoacidosis and a hypoglycemic reaction by completing the following chart:

	Hypoglycemia (insulin reaction)	Hyperglycemia (keto-acidosis)
Onset	a.	b.
Cause	c.	d.
Manifestations	e.	f.
Ominous features	g.	h.
Urinary findings	i.	j.
Blood glucose	k.	l.

46. Insulin injections are rotated to various parts of the body. What is the rationale for this action?

47. The appropriate emergency measure when a diabetic child is having a hypoglycemic reaction is to administer _____ in some form.

48. Compliance to the diabetic regimen is sometimes a problem, especially in the _____ age group.

IV. Application, Analysis, and Synthesis of Essential Concepts

A. Experiential Exercise: Spend a day in a pediatric endocrine clinic. Answer the following questions and include specific examples or responses to illustrate these concepts.

1. List the clinical manifestations you would expect to assess in a child with hypopituitarism.
   a.

   b.

   c.

   d.

   e.

   f.

   g.

   h.

2. List the clinical manifestations you would expect to assess in a child with hyperpituitarism before epiphyseal closure.
   a.

   b.

   c.

   d.

3. List the clinical manifestations you would expect to assess in an infant with diabetes insipidus.

a.

b.

c.

d.

4. What piece of assessment data would alert you to the possibility of an infant having hypothyroidism?

5. The primary nursing goal in relation to hypothyroidism is:

6. Nursing interventions to achieve the nursing goal of "maintaining the safety of the patient" in a patient experiencing a deficiency in parathyroid would be:
a.

b.

c.

d.

B. Experiential Exercise: Care for a child with adrenocortical insufficiency. Answer the following questions and include specifics (examples, responses) to illustrate these concepts.
1. You would take the child's vital signs every 15 minutes. What is the rationale for this intervention?

2. When administering cortisol to the child, the nurse carefully checks the dosage and the rate of administration. What is the rationale for these actions?

3. As treatment progresses, you continually assess the child for signs of hypokalemia. What are these signs?

C. Experiential Exercise: Care for a child with the salt-losing form of congenital adrenogenital hyperplasia.
1. A primary nursing goal in relation to the child with adrenogenital hyperplasia is:

2. The rationale for administering cortisone to the child with adrenogenital syndrome is:

D. Clinical Situation: Bobby Lee Jones, an 8-year-old, is on the pediatric unit for diagnosis and treatment of diabetes mellitus.
1. When Bobby arrived on the unit, he was displaying symptoms of ketoacidosis.
   a. What are the four goals for the management of Bobby's care?
   1)

   2)

   3)

   4)

   b. What evaluation data would you expect for the nursing goal of "Ensure adequate hydration"?

2. Bobby is placed on NPH insulin twice a day. The nurse must intervene by monitoring whether the insulin dose is appropriate. What is the best method to do this?

3. Bobby will be maintained on a balanced diet employing the exchange system of the American Diabetic Association. The nursing goal regarding this diet is to:

4. Bobby is experiencing a hypoglycemic reaction.
   a. What symptoms would you expect to assess in Bobby?

   b. How would you intervene to treat the hypoglycemia?

5. What are the overall nursing goals for a child like Bobby?
   a.

   b.

   c.

   d.

6. What evaluative data would give evidence of the accomplishment of the goal of "Nurse will facilitate self-management"?

E. Experiential Exercise: Design a teaching plan for the child with diabetes mellitus.
  1. What nursing goals are appropriate to include in this teaching plan?
  a.

  b.

  c.

  d.

  e.

  f.

  g.

  h.

  i.

  j.

  k.

  l.

V. Suggested Readings

Frey MA, Fox MA: Assessing and teaching self-care to youths with diabetes mellitus, Pediatr Nurs 16(6):597-599, 1990.

> The purpose of this research was "to investigate the nature of diabetes self-care in youths with IDDM and to relate diabetes self-care to metabolic control, perceived health status, and general (universal) self-care." The study included 37 youths between the ages of 11 and 19. The results showed that diabetes self-care was positively related to general self-care, health status, and metabolic control. Implications for nursing practice are explored.

Hahn K: Teaching patients to administer insulin, Nursing 90 90(4):70, 1990.

> This article is an illustrated explanation of the do's and don'ts of insulin administration that is essential to patient teaching.

McElroy D, Davis G: SIADH and the acutely ill child, Am J Maternal Child Nurs 11:193-196, 1986.

> This thorough discussion of SIADH covers the pathophysiology, detection, and treatment of this complex disease.

Chapter 29

The Child with Integumentary Dysfunction

I.   Chapter Overview

Chapter 29 introduces the various disorders that affect the skin, the largest organ in the body. Alterations in the integrity of the skin caused by bacterial, viral, and fungal infections; environmental and internal antigens; stings and bites; or thermal injury are explored. Content is presented to familiarize the student with the manifestations in the skin caused by these disorders. The supportive and curative nursing interventions common to these disorders are discussed. The knowledge gained in this chapter will help the student formulate an effective care plan for the child with an alteration in skin integrity.

II. Learning Objectives

Upon completion of this chapter, it is expected that the student will be able to:

1.   Describe the distribution and configuration of the various skin lesions.

2.   List the benefits of a moist environment for wound healing.

3.   Discuss the nursing care related to therapies for skin disorders.

4.   Contrast the manifestations of and therapies for bacterial, viral, and fungal infections of the skin.

5.   Compare the skin manifestations related to age in children.

6.   Outline a plan of care to prevent and treat diaper dermatitis.

7.   Outline a plan of care for a child with atopic dermatitis.

8.   Formulate a teaching plan for an adolescent with acne.

9.   Describe the methods for assessing a burn wound.

10.   Discuss the physical and emotional care of a child with a severe burn wound.

III. Review of Essential Concepts

1.   ____ The skin is the largest organ in the body. (true or false)

2.   Identify the four functions of the skin.
      a.

      b.

      c.

      d.

3.   List the three general etiologic factors related to skin lesions.
      a.

      b.

      c.

4. Match the following terms used to describe skin lesions with their correct definitions.
   a. ___ erythema
   b. ___ ecchymoses
   c. ___ petechiae
   d. ___ primary lesions
   e. ___ secondary lesions
      1) pinpoint tiny and sharply circumscribed spots in the superficial layers of the epidermis
      2) localized red or purple discolorations caused by extravasation of blood into the dermis and subcutaneous tissues
      3) changes that result from alteration in a lesion, such as those caused by rubbing
      4) a reddened area caused by increased amounts of oxygenated blood in the dermal vasculature
      5) skin changes produced by some causative factor

5. Wounds are defined as:

6. Wounds are classified as:
   a.

   b.

   c.

7. The mechanism of wound healing with scar formation involves the processes of:
   a.

   b.

   c.

   d.

8. The safest solution to apply to wounds is _____.

9. The major goals of therapeutic management in wound healing are:
   a.

   b.

   c.

   d.

10. List the functions that dressings serve:

11. Identify the three categories of occlusive dressings.
    a.

    b.

    c.

12. The nurse should teach parents that hydrocortisone preparations:
    a. can be used for all skin disorders
    b. should be applied as a heavy coating
    c. should be massaged into the skin in a thin layer
    d. can be used only for short periods

13. Signs of wound infection are:

14. The nursing goals of care for the child with a skin condition are:
    a.

    b.

    c.

    d.

15. Most of the therapeutic regimens in caring for disorders of the skin are directed toward relief of _____.

16. Wet compresses or dressings provide the following purposes:

17. When taking a bath, use a solution of _____ or _____.

18. ___ The incidence of staphylococcal infections in children increases with advancing age. (true or false)

19. The two major nursing goals related to bacterial skin infections are:
    a.

    b.

20. When a child is admitted to the hospital with cellulitis, nursing interventions include:
    a.

b.

c.

21. In what two ways do epidermal cells react to viral infection?
a.

b.

22. Dermatophytoses (ringworm) are treated with the drug _____ or _____ for a period of weeks or months.
23. Define *contact dermatitis*.

24. The major nursing goal in the care of the child with contact dermatitis is to:

25. ___ A nursing intervention following known contact with a poisonous plant is to immediately help the child scrub the affected area with hot, soapy water. (true or false)
26. The organ in which adverse drug reactions are most often seen is the:
a. liver
b. kidney
c. bone marrow
d. skin
27. Describe the nurse's responsibility when a rash is suspected to represent a drug reaction.

28. The skin infestations encountered most frequently in childhood are _____ and _____.
29. List the four areas of the child's body that the nurse should be particularly careful to assess for scabies lesions.
a.

b.

c.

d.

30. Scabies is treated by the application of _____.
31. In teaching parents about pediculosis capitis, the nurse should emphasize that:
a. head lice are carried by household pets
b. lice can be transmitted on personal items
c. cleanliness is the best protection against lice
d. cutting the child's hair prevents reinfestation
32. Children who are hypersensitive to insect bites or stings are treated with _____.
33. ___ Cat scratch disease is a benign, self-limiting illness that resolves spontaneously in 2 to 4 months. (true or false)
34. The most common contact dermatitis in infants occurs on the convex surfaces of the diaper area as a result of irritation from:

35. The aims of nursing management for diaper dermatitis are to:
a.

b.

c.

36. Match the skin disorders on the right with their clinical manifestations on the left.
a. ___ appears on scalp, face, arms, and legs; lesions are red, have papules and vesicles, and are itchy
b. ___ appears on the scalp, eyelids, and external ear canal; lesions are thick, yellowish, and scaly
c. ___ appears on convex surfaces or in skin folds
   1) seborrheic dermatitis
   2) atopic dermatitis
   3) diaper dermatitis
37. List the measures used in the therapeutic management of eczema.
a.

b.

c.

d.

38. Seborrheic dermatitis is:

39. The skin disorder that appears predominantly during the adolescent period is _____.

40. The statement that correctly describes acne is:
   a. The peak incidence of acne is during the period of middle childhood.
   b. Lesions seen in acne may be either noninflamed comedones or inflamed lesions.
   c. The pathogenesis of acne is related to an abnormality of the sebaceous glands.
   d. Primary inflammation in acne is usually caused by the presence of *Staphylococcus albus*.

41. The most effective therapy for acne involves the use of _____, or _____, or a combination of the two drugs.

42. What are the three factors considered in assessing the severity of a burn?
   a.

   b.

   c.

43. A characteristic of a superficial burn is:
   a. absence of pain
   b. major tissue damage
   c. systemic effects
   d. frequently, a latent period followed by erythema

44. A systemic response to a thermal injury would include:
   a. decreased metabolic rate
   b. decreased urine output
   c. hypoglycemia
   d. hypertension

45. Why is anemia often seen in patients with a burn injury?

46. The immediate threat to life following a thermal injury is _____.

47. The aims of the immediate treatment of a thermal injury are:
   a.

   b.

   c.

   d.

   e.

48. The primary concerns of therapeutic management are:
   a.

   b.

   c.

49. The objectives of fluid replacement for the child with burns are:
   a.

   b.

   c.

   d.

   e.

   f.

50. The early surgical excision of eschar in deep partial-thickness and full-thickness burns has reduced _____ _____.

51. Differentiate between open and closed dressing for burns.
   a. Open–

   b. Closed–

52. A homograft is:

53. The goals of nursing care for the burned child are:
   a.

   b.

   c.

   d.

   e.

   f.

   g.

   h.

54. Signs and symptoms of sepsis associated with burns are:

55. _____ from sunburn is the major goal of medical and nursing management.

56. ___ Sunscreens are recommended for infants less than 6 months of age. (true or false)

57. Frostbite results from:

IV. Application, Analysis, and Synthesis of Essential Concepts

A. Experiential Exercise: Care for a hospitalized child with a skin disorder. Answer the following questions and include specific examples to illustrate these concepts.

  1. Develop five nursing diagnoses that would be appropriate for a child with a skin disorder.
  a.

  b.

  c.

  d.

  e.

  2. Provide the rationale for each of the following nursing interventions that may be used in the care of the child with a skin disorder.
  a. Administer soaks, baths, or lotions–

  b. Apply topical corticosteroids to affected area–

  c. Employ restraint devices and scrupulous hygiene–

  d. Apply intermittent wet dressings–

  e. Apply occlusive dressings–

B. Clinical Situation: A home visit has been scheduled to assist Mrs. Stone in caring for her 5-month-old infant, Andrew, who has atopic dermatitis. The infant is also suspected of having cow's milk sensitivity.

  1. The principal nursing objective in caring for the child with cow's milk sensitivity is:

  2. Formulate at least three nursing diagnoses that pertain to the child who has eczema:
  a.

  b.

  c.

  3. The nursing goal for the nursing diagnosis of "impaired skin integrity related to environmental agents, somatic factors, immunologic deficit" is:

C. Clinical Situation: Mrs. Ryan brings 2-month-old Sean to the clinic for his well-child visit. Upon examination you discover that Sean has severe diaper dermatitis.

  1. How was the diagnosis of diaper dermatitis made?

2. Nursing interventions for diaper dermatitis are aimed at altering _____.

3. What interventions might you suggest to Mrs. Ryan to treat and prevent the diaper rash?

   a.

   b.

   c.

   d.

   e.

D. Clinical Situation: Lester Robitaille, age 9 years, is brought to the pediatric health center by his mother. She states that Lester has been scratching his head and she has found small white specks in his hair. Mrs. Robitaille brings a note from the school stating that head lice have been found in several children in Lester's classroom.

1. Why are schoolchildren highly susceptible to communicable diseases, including infestations?

2. What causes the characteristic itching seen with pediculosis?

3. _____ is the drug of choice in the treatment of pediculosis.

4. What two types of programs must accompany the treatment of pediculosis for it to be effective?

   a.

   b.

5. What is the rationale for reapplying the pediculicide 7 to 10 days after the initial treatment?

E. Experiential Exercise: Care for a child who has sustained a thermal injury.

1. What interventions prevent fluid overload?

   a.

   b.

   c.

2. How do you evaluate the success of the interventions in maintaining your patient's renal function?

3. What is the rationale for wearing sterile gowns, masks, and gloves while in the patient's room?

4. You notice that your patient is not eating all of the food on the plate. Formulate one nursing diagnosis that reflects this observation.

5. What is the rationale for monitoring the patient's bowel function?

6. How do you evaluate whether the nursing goal of preparing the family for discharge is accomplished?

V. Suggested Readings

Deitch EA, editor: The management of burns, Engl J Med 323(18):1249-1253, 1990.

   The goal of this review was to present an overview of the principles of care of patients with burns. The areas of focus are cardiopulmonary resuscitation, metabolism and nutrition, infection and immunity, and therapy of the burn wound.

Farrington E, editor: Diaper dermatitis, Pediatr Nurs 18(1):81-82, 1992.

   A concise exploration of types of diaper dermatitis, etiology, complications, and prevention and treatment. A table of over-the-counter compounds is a useful addendum.

Willey T: Use a decision tree to choose wound dressings, Am J Nurs 92(2):43-46, 1992.

> According to the author, more than 2000 products are available to aid wound healing. A unique resource, a decision tree, is included to enable nurses to combine careful wound assessment with selection of an appropriate dressing. The decision tree aids nurses by combining their assessment with a specialist's knowledge of wound dressing products.

Wong D, and others: Diapering choices: a critical review of the issues, Pediatr Nurs 18(1):41-54, 1992.

> This is a critical review of the issues related to cloth versus disposable paper diapers. The diapering systems were compared on five variables: skin care, infection control, other health care considerations, environmental and safety concerns, and time/cost issues. This is a thorough exploration of this topic firmly grounded on research.

Chapter 30

The Child with Musculoskeletal or Articular Dysfunction

I. Chapter Overview

Chapter 30 introduces nursing considerations to the care of the child immobilized with an injury or a degenerative disease. The disorders considered are of congenital, acquired, traumatic, infectious, neoplastic, or idiopathic origin. The conditions may be either temporary or permanent; however, they all affect the child's locomotive ability to a greater or lesser extent. Nursing goals and responsibilities are developed to help the child and family effectively cope with the physical, emotional, and psychosocial stressors imposed by impaired mobility.

II. Learning Objectives

Upon completion of this chapter, it is expected that the student will be able to:

1. Outline a plan for the care of a child immobilized with an injury or a degenerative disease.

2. Formulate a teaching plan for the parents of a child in a cast.

3. Explain the functions of the various types of traction.

4. Devise a nursing care plan for a child in traction.

5. Differentiate among the various congenital skeletal defects.

6. Design a teaching plan for the parents of a child with a congenital skeletal deformity.

7. Describe the therapies and nursing care of a child with scoliosis.

8. Outline a plan of care for the child with osteomyelitis.

9. Differentiate between osteosarcoma and Ewing sarcoma.

10. Describe the nursing care of a child with juvenile rheumatoid arthritis.

11. Demonstrate an understanding of the management of systemic lupus erythematosus.

III. Review of Essential Concepts

1. List the consequences of immobilization of the child.
   a.

   b.

   c.

2. The psychological and emotional consequences of immobilization to the child can severely affect normal growth and development. One of the most useful interventions to help children cope with immobility is to encourage the child to _____
_____.

3. Define the following traumatic injuries:
   a. Contusion–

   b. Dislocation–

   c. Sprain–

   d. Strain–

4. In the first 6 to 12 hours of injury, the basic principles of managing soft tissue injuries are represented by RICE. Explain:
   a. R =

   b. I =

   c. C =

   d. E =

5. List and describe the most commonly seen fractures in children.
   a.

   b.

   c.

   d.

6. The three goals of therapeutic management are:
   a.

   b.

   c.

7. In children, the bone fragments are usually realigned and immobilized by _____ or by _____ and _____ until adequate callus is formed.

8. During the first few hours after a cast is applied, the nurse must observe the cast and the involved extremity for signs of neurovascular integrity. What signs would indicate compromise in the extremity?

9. What are the three primary purposes for use of traction for reduction of fractures?
   a.

   b.

   c.

10. What are the three methods of applying pull to the distal bone fragment for traction?
    a.

    b.

    c.

11. Compare the functions of the various types of traction for the lower extremity by matching the following:
    1) Balance suspension
    2) 90°-90° traction
    3) Buck's extension
    4) Russell traction
    5) Bryant's traction
    a. ____ A form of running traction used for children less than 2 years of age
    b. ____ A form of running traction in which hips are not flexed
    c. ____ A form of skin traction that has two lines of pull, one along the longitudinal line of the lower leg and one perpendicular to the leg
    d. ____ Lower leg is put in a boot cast, and a skeletal Steinmann pin is placed in the distal fragment of the femur
    e. ____ The leg is suspended in a desired flexed position to relax the hip and hamstring muscles; no traction is exerted directly on a body part

12. When amputated, a severed part should be preserved in what manner to facilitate reattachment?

13. List the three degrees of congenital hip dysplasia.
a.

b.

c.

14. In the child between birth and 2 months of age, subluxation and the tendency to dislocate are most reliably demonstrated by the _____ and _____ tests.

15. Match the following types of club foot positions with their defining characteristics.
a. ___ talipes varus
b. ___ talipes equinus
c. ___ talipes valgus
d. ___ talipes calceneus
1) plantar flexion in which the toes are lower than the heel
2) an eversion or bending outward
3) dorsiflexion, in which the toes are higher than the heel
4) an inversion or bending inward

16. Therapeutic management of congenital club foot involves:
a.

b.

c.

17. Osteogenesis imperfecta is a group of _____ of connective tissue characterized by _____ tissue and bone defects.

18. List the four stages of Legg-Calve-Perthes disease:
a. Stage I–

b. Stage II–

c. Stage III–

d. Stage IV–

19. What are the two classifications of scoliosis?
a.

b.

20. Scoliosis is currently managed by straightening and realignment of the vertebrae by either:

21. _____ is the primary mode of therapy for minor curvatures.

22. _____ is often used before spinal fusion to provide partial correction and more flexibility.

23. Following Harrington instrumentation the child is immobilized on a _____ _____. Children with Dwyer instrumentation are cared for in _____.

24. What is the primary advantage and disadvantage of the Lugue segmental instrumentation?

25. Osteomyelitis is an _____ _____, which can be acquired from _____ or _____ sources.

26. When the infective agent of osteomyelitis is identified, vigorous _____ is initiated with an appropriate _____.

27. In addition to antibiotic therapy the child with osteomyelitis is placed on _____ and the affected extremity is _____ _____.

28. Tubercular extension of infection to other sites in children is usually to the _____ or _____.

29. In children two types of bone tumors that account for 85% of all primary malignant bone tumors are _____ and _____.

30. Compare osteogenic sarcoma and Ewing sarcoma in terms of etiology and therapeutic management.

	Osteogenic Sarcoma	Ewing Sarcoma
Etiology	a.	b.
Management	c.	d.

31. If an amputation is performed for osteogenic sarcoma, the child is usually fitted with a temporary _____ immediately after surgery.

32. The latex fixation text is diagnostic for rheumatoid arthritis in the adult. In children the latex fixation test is _____.

33. What are the clinical manifestations of juvenile rheumatoid arthritis (JRA)?

34. Growth disturbances are often present in the child with JRA. What are the reasons?
    a.

    b.

35. What are the major goals of therapy for the child with JRA?
    a.

    b.

    c.

36. The primary groups of drugs prescribed for JRA are:
    a.

    b.

    c.

    d.

37. Why are corticosteroids not a drug of choice for JRA?

38. Systemic lupus erythematosus (SLE) is:

39. SLE can affect almost any tissue, so the clinical manifestations vary according to the tissue affected. However, a characteristic cutaneous response of SLE is:

40. Identify the gravest prognostic sign in SLE.

41. Identify the objectives of therapeutic management of SLE.
    a.

    b.

42. Identify the principal drugs employed to control the inflammation of SLE.

43. Identify the principal nursing goal for the child with SLE.

44. Identify the relationship of rest to the status of SLE.

IV. Application, Analysis, and Synthesis of Essential Concepts

A. Experiential Exercise: Spend a day on the neurologic unit observing the care of immobilized children. The nurse must plan the care of the immobilized child with the knowledge that immobilization causes functional and metabolic responses in most of the body systems.

1. Identify the nursing diagnoses appropriate for the care of the immobilized child.
    a.

    b.

    c.

    d.

    e.

2. General nursing goals for the immobilized child are:
    a.

    b.

    c.

    d.

3. What manifestations of tissue ischemia of the skin would you assess to detect skin breakdown?

B. Experiential Exercise: Spend a day on a pediatric orthopedic unit.
1. A 5-year-old child with a fractured right leg has just had a cast applied. The nurse must intervene by teaching the parents how to care for the cast. What elements would you include in your teaching plan regarding methods to decrease the swelling under the cast?
   a.

   b.

   c.

   d.

2. What elements would you include in a teaching plan regarding maintaining the integrity of the cast?
   a.

   b.

   c.

C. Clinical Situation: Roger Trudeau, age 13 years, is in 90-degree-90-degree traction for treatment of a fracture of the right femur.
1. Identify the nursing interventions that will achieve the nursing goal of "maintaining the traction."
   a.

   b.

   c.

   d.

   e.

   f.

   g.

2. Identify a nursing diagnosis in which the primary nursing goal is "prevent complications."

3. You would assess the Steinmann pin for signs of _____ or _____ _____ or for _____ to detect problems.

D. Experiential Exercise: Care for a child with congenital hip dysplasia.
1. During the infant assessment process, what clinical signs could indicate congenital dislocation of the hip in the newborn?
   a.

   b.

   c.

   d.

   e.

2. Therapeutic treatment is begun as _____ as possible, and will vary according to the _____ of the child and the extent of the _____.
3. The goals of nursing care when preparing the child and parents for discharge are:
   a.

   b.

   c.

4. What instructions should be incorporated into a teaching plan for the parents of a child who is being discharged with a reduction appliance such as a Pavlik harness?
   a.

   b.

   c.

   d.

   e.

f.

g.

E. Clinical Situation: Jane Roberts, age 14 years, is admitted to the adolescent unit with a diagnosis of scoliosis. She is being prepared for a Lugue segmental instrumentation.
   1. What is an important nursing diagnosis that may be evidence when the nurse considers the interaction of Jane's physical defect and psychological growth and developmental processes of the adolescent?
      a.

      or:
      b.

   2. What nursing interventions are appropriate to promote the nursing goal of "Help the child develop a positive self-image"?
      a.

      b.

      c.

      d.

   3. To control the pain after surgery what would be the most appropriate choice of drug and method of administration?

F. Clinical Situation: Emmanuel Rogerio, age 10 years, is admitted for treatment of osteomyelitis.
   1. What clinical manifestations would you expect to assess in Emmanuel if the diagnosis is correct?

   2. What nursing interventions are appropriate for the nursing goal of "Maintain intravenous infusion"?
      a.

b.

c.

d.

G. Clinical Situation: Robin Monteira, age 11 years, is admitted to the pediatric unit for treatment of JRA.
   1. Identify evaluation data that would indicate accomplishment of the nursing goal of "Prevent physical deformity and preserve joint function."

   2. Identify an appropriate nursing diagnosis related to nutrition in Robin.

   3. Since Robin is on high doses of aspirin, you would assess for aspirin toxicity. Identify the signs of aspirin toxicity and their underlying etiology.
      a.

      b.

      c.

      d.

V. **Suggested Readings**

Olson V: The hazards of immobility, Am J Nurs 90(3):43-48, 1990.

This is a reprint of the classic article first published in 1967. Only two sections (Effects on Cardiovascular Function, Effects on Respiratory Function) are included. This article remains an authoritative reference in the care of the bedbound patient, and is an essential reference for the effective nurse.

Redheffer GM, Bailey M: Assessing and splinting fractures, Nursing 89 89(6):51-59, 1989.

The focus of this article is to enable the nurse to assess and to immobilize a fracture of the leg, wrist, clavicle, or humerus. A step-by-step guide, complete with photographs, clearly illustrates the content.

Southwood TR, and others: Unconventional remedies used for patients with juvenile arthritis, Pediatrics 85(2):150-153, 1990.

Fifty-three patients with juvenile arthritis from Australia, New Zealand, and Canada completed questionnaires while attending an arthritis youth camp. More than 70% of the respondents admitted using unconventional remedies. The most commonly used unconventional remedies were copper bracelets, diet, and patent medicines. The potential dangers of unconventional remedies are explored, and professionals are warned to consider this possibility when working with this type of patient.

Wise LB: A comparison of orthopedic casts: breaking the mold, Am J Maternal Child Nurs 11:174-176, 1986.

The author compares the plaster-of-paris cast and the synthetic casts on five parameters. General nursing goals and nursing care considerations for care of the child in a cast are introduced.

Chapter 31

The Child with Neuromuscular or Muscular Dysfunction

I. Chapter Overview

Chapter 31 introduces nursing considerations essential to the care of the child with a disorder of neuromuscular function. Since childhood is the age of onset for a variety of physically disabling conditions, it is important for the student to gain an understanding of the care of children with this type of alteration in health. The conditions discussed in this chapter may result from defective transmission of nerve impulses to muscles, dysfunction of peripheral motor or sensory nerves, or damage to the central nervous system. At the completion of this chapter, the student will be able to formulate nursing measures directed toward helping the child and his family develop effective coping responses to deal with alterations in neuromuscular function.

II. Learning Objectives

Upon completion of this chapter, it is expected that the student will be able to:

1. Discuss the nursing role in helping parents cope with a child with cerebral palsy.

2. Formulate a nursing care plan for the preoperative and postoperative care of the child with myelomeningocele.

3. Outline a plan of care for a child with Duchenne muscular dystrophy.

4. Identify the causes of botulism in infants and children.

5. List three causes of spinal cord injury in children.

6. Discuss the prevention and treatment of tetanus.

III. Review of Essential Concepts

1. Cerebral palsy is:

2. Is there a characteristic pathologic picture of cerebral palsy?

3. List and define the classifications of cerebral palsy.
   a.

   b.

   c.

   d.

   e.

4. The clinical manifestations of cerebral palsy fall into five major areas. What are they?

a.

b.

c.

d.

e.

5. What is the relationship between cerebral palsy and mental retardation?

6. The broad aims of therapy for the child with cerebral palsy are:

a.

b.

c.

d.

7. The most frequently employed conservative treatment modality is _____.

8. _____ refers to a hernial protrusion of a saclike cyst containing meninges, spinal fluid, and a portion of the spinal cord with its nerves through a defect in the vertebral column.
a. Rachischisis
b. Meningocele
c. Encephalocele
d. Myelomeningocele

9. An important nursing intervention when caring for a child with a myelomeningocele in the preoperative stage would be:
a. applying a heat lamp to facilitate drying and toughening of the sac
b. assessing sensory and motor function frequently to monitor for signs of impairment
c. applying a diaper to prevent contamination of the sac
d. placing the child on his side to decrease pressure on the spinal cord

10. All of the muscular dystrophies have a genetic origin in which there is a gradual degeneration of _____, and all are characterized by _____ _____.

11. In all forms of muscular dystrophy there is insidious loss of strength; the various forms differ in regard to:

12. The most severe and most common muscular dystrophy of childhood is:

13. The cause of death in Duchenne muscular dystrophy is:

14. _____ involving large and small joints compromise mobility.

15. The primary goal of therapy is:

16. Guillain-Barré syndrome is an:

17. Treatment of Guillain-Barré syndrome is symptomatic, but _____ may be needed to preserve life.

18. Tetanus is:

19. The characteristic symptom of tetanus that gives the disease its common name of lockjaw is:

20. Preventive measures for tetanus are based on the _____ of the affected child and the nature of the _____.

21. The unimmunized child who sustains a "tetanus-prone" wound should receive _____.

22. What specific nursing interventions are employed to prevent seizures in the child with tetanus?

   a.

   b.

23. Infant botulism is caused by:

24. Although inadequately cooked or improperly canned food is the prime source of botulism, the organism has been found in _____ and _____ added to infant formulas as sweeteners.

25. Diagnosis of botulism is based on:

26. With spinal cord injury, the higher the injury the more extensive the damage. Two terms that are used to describe such damage are paraplegia and quadriplegia. Define these terms.

   a. Paraplegia =

   b. Quadriplegia =

IV. Application, Analysis, and Synthesis of Essential Concepts

A. Experiential Exercise: Spend a day in a clinic that treats children with cerebral palsy.
   1. What specific nursing goals would help the parents and child with cerebral palsy?
      a.

      b.

      c.

      d.

      e.

      f.

2. List at least two nursing diagnoses for a child with cerebral palsy.
   a.

   b.

B. Clinical Situation: Adam McElroy, a newborn, is transferred to the pediatric unit for surgical evaluation of a myelomeningocele.
   1. Identify three nursing goals for Adam's initial care.
      a.

      b.

      c.

   2. What evaluative data would indicate the accomplishment of each of the above nursing goals?
      a.

      b.

      c.

C. Experiential Exercise: Spend a day in a clinic serving children with muscular dystrophy.
   1. Because parents of children with muscular dystrophy tend to overprotect their child, how would you intervene to assist both child and family?

   2. Because of the genetic etiology of this disease, you would intervene by:

D. Clinical Situation: Victor Morris, age 13 years, has been admitted to the pediatric unit with a diagnosis of Guillain-Barre syndrome.
   1. The primary nursing goal is:

   2. List at least two nursing interventions to achieve the above nursing goal.
      a.

      b.

E. Clinical Situation: Anthonio Ruiz, age 15 years, is hospitalized in a rehabilitation center for treatment of paraplegia caused by a spinal cord injury.

1. The primary nursing goals for care of Antonio in the acute period are:

   a.

   b.

2. Although nursing involvement is essential to the care of Antonio, to be truly effective the plan of care must be carried out by an _____ team.

V. Suggested Readings

Birdsall C: How do you teach female self-catheterization? Am J Nurs 85:1226-1227, 1985.

> The variables that the nurse must consider when teaching self-catheterization are outlined. A step-by-step procedure for performing the self-catheterization is included.

Chadwick AT, Oesting HH: Caring for patients with spinal cord injuries. Nursing 89 89(11):52-56, 1989.

> This article provides a complete overview of the care of the patient with a spinal cord injury. The aspects explored are type of injury, skin care, respiratory care, bladder care, minimizing infection risks, bowel care, and aiding mobility and transfers. A helpful table summarizes how the level of spinal injury affects daily activities.

Lancaster MJ: Botulism: north to Alaska, 90(1):60-62, 1990.

> This article is primarily concerned with the rising incidence of botulism in the state of Alaska, but the discussion of the assessment, diagnosis, and medical and nursing care of the affected client is universally applicable information.

Romeo JH: Spinal cord injury: nursing the patient toward a new life, RN 88(5):31-35, 1988.

> The care of the newly injured spinal cord patient is discussed. The author traces nursing care and planning from emergency admission to discharge. Prevention of complications is a primary focus.

Answer Key

Chapter 1

Question   Answer

Section III

1. 21
2. Japan
3. low birthweight
4. injuries (accidents)
5. sex and age
6. a
7. b
8. b
9. new morbidity
10. financial barriers; system barriers; knowledge barriers
11. primary nursing
12.
    a. family advocacy
    b. illness prevention and health promotion
    c. health teaching
    d. support and counseling
    e. therapeutic role
    f. coordination and collaboration
    g. research
    h. health care planning
13. therapeutic relationship

Section IV A

1.
    a. the number of individuals who have died over a specific period of time
    b. the prevalence of a specific illness in the population at a particular time
2. Knowledge of these two concepts can help identify high-risk age groups for certain disorders, identify advances in prevention and treatment, direct energies into specific areas of health counseling, and guide more effective planning and delivery of care.
3. The most effective approach to reducing morbidity and mortality is through the nurse's role in educating parents and promoting optimum health practices.

Section IV B

1.
    a. Ensure families' awareness of various health services; inform families of treatments and procedures; involve families in child's care; change or support existing health care practices.
    b. Practice within the overall framework for preventive health; employ an approach of education and anticipatory guidance.
    c. Provide health education and evaluate the status of and need for health knowledge.
    d. Provide support through listening, touching, and physical presence; use counseling as the basis for mutual problem solving.
    e. Continual assessment and evaluation of the health status of client; a therapeutic relationship is essential to fulfilling all aspects of the therapeutic role.

f. Work with professionals in other disciplines to formulate and implement a plan of care that meets the child's needs.

g. Conduct research to provide theoretical foundations for nursing practice and to evaluate the nursing process.

h. Become involved in policy and decision-making on the community and national levels to enhance health care delivery.

2. Primary nursing involves 24-hour responsibility and accountability for the care of a small group of patients. In this capacity, nurses are responsible for their actions, in both the legal and ethical sense. If the nurse's responsibilities are shared with other staff, it is usually with an associate primary nurse who maintains continuity of care and assumes only temporary accountability.

Chapter 2

Question   Answer

Section III

1.
  a. assessment
  b. nursing diagnosis
  c. planning
  d. implementation
  e. evaluation

2.
  a. Thorough assessment of child and family.
  b. Answers to selected questions from each area obtained to determine if more information is needed.
  c. In-depth assessment performed in a particular area when screening assessment indicates problem may exist.

3. 11; functional health patterns

4.
  a. Health perception-health management pattern
  b. Nutritional-Metabolic Pattern
  c. Elimination Pattern
  d. Activity-Exercise Pattern
  e. Sleep-Rest Pattern
  f. Self-Perception, Self-Concept Pattern
  g. Role-Relationship Pattern
  h. Sexuality-Reproductive Pattern
  i. Coping-Stress Tolerance Pattern
  j. Value-Belief Pattern
  k. Cognitive-Perceptual Pattern

5.
  a. Dependent activities — areas of nursing practice that hold the nurse accountable for implementing the prescribed medical regimen.

b. Interdependent activities — areas of nursing practice in which medical and nursing responsibility and accountability overlap and require collaboration between the two disciplines.

c. Independent activities — areas of nursing practice that are the direct responsibility of the nurse.

6. Interdependent; independent

7. Problem; etiology; signs and symptoms

8.
  a. 1
  b. 3
  c. 2

9. outcomes, goals

10.
  a. Focus on the problem statement of the nursing diagnosis.
  b. Using measurable verbs describe the desired patient's behavior or change in clinical status.
  c. Add modifiers that describe what, where, how, and when.
  d. Add the achievement time.
  e. Examine the statement. Determine if it is measurable, realistic, and achievable.

11.
  a. Plans that are sufficiently broad to account for situations that may develop in patients with particular problems.
  b. Plans that are concerned with only those diagnoses that apply to the particular patient situation.

12. The actual delivery of nursing care to the patient using the nursing and medical plans of care.

13. evaluation

Section IV A

1.
  a. Interview/health history; child, family, significant individuals
  b. Observation of social interactions
  c. Developmental assessment
  d. Physical assessment
  e. Laboratory data
  f. Consultation with other health professionals

2.
  a. Cognitive-Perceptual Pattern
  b. Pain related to abdominal incision
  c. Pain
  d. Abdominal incision
  e. Inability to lie comfortably in a supine position

3. Client will be able to lie in a supine position without pain within 48 hours.

4. Administer pain medication as ordered.

5. Client is able to lie in supine position without discomfort.

Section IV B

1. Individualized
2. Standardized
3. Individualized
4. Individualized
5. Standardized

Chapter 3

Question   Answer

Section III

1.
   a. 2
   b. 4
   c. 3
   d. 1
2.
   a. intimate, continued face-to-face contact, mutual support of the members, and the ability to order or constrain a considerable proportion of individual members' behavior
   b. groups that have limited intermittent contact and in which there is generally less concern for members' behavior
3. ethnicity, social class, occupational role
4. The classification of or affiliation with any of the basic groups or divisions of mankind or any heterogeneous population differentiated by customs, characteristics, language or similar distinguishing factors.
5. social class
6.
   a. Parents value the concrete and tangible rather than the abstract and are therefore less inclined to encourage these qualities in their children.
   b. Parents are less likely to read to the child or encourage educational play due to their own educational level.
   c. No role models may be available to support the value of education.
   d. Inadequate funding and/or poor quality of education exists in neighborhood schools.
   e. Poor health and inadequate nutrition of the children is common.
   f. Limited communication skills, such as simple grammar, inability to express

abstractions, and ethnic dialects that hamper interactions with teachers from middle-class backgrounds.
7. lack of money or material resources, which includes insufficient clothing, poor sanitation, and deteriorating housing
8. social and cultural deprivation such as limited employment opportunities, inferior educational opportunities, lack of or inferior medical services and health care facilities, and an absence of public services
9. preschool
10. migrant
11.
   a. teaches the child how to deal with dominance and hostility
   b. teaches the children to relate with persons in positions of leadership and authority
   c. relieves the child's boredom
   d. provides recognition that individual members do not receive from teachers and other authority figures
12. optimism; geographic; economic input; role; nuclear; neighborhoods
13. the "feelings of helplessness and discomfort and a state of disorientation experienced by an outsider attempting to comprehend or effectively adapt to a different cultural group because of differences in cultural practices, values, and beliefs"
14.
   a. 4
   b. 1
   c. 3
   d. 2
15. values; beliefs, customs
16. cultural relativity
17.
   a. attitude toward time and waiting
   b. person responsible for health care
   c. manner of approach to child
   d. family involvement
   e. tension with members of majority group
   f. verbal and nonverbal communication
   g. level of comfort with body space or distance or distance from others
   h. eye contact
   i. ability to question
   j. terms of address
   k. expression of emotion
   l. food customs
   m. health beliefs
   n. health practices
18.
   a. Church of Christ Scientist
   b. Jehovah's Witness
   c. Roman Catholic

Section IV A

1. The culture in which children are reared determines the types of food they will eat, the language they will speak, the ideals of behavior, and the way in which social roles should be conducted. It also outlines the roles of their parents, structures their relationships with other people, and determines much of the behavior they acquire.

2.
   a. ethnicity
   b. social class
   c. economic status
   d. occupation
   e. religion
   f. education
   g. peer influences

3.
   a. results in a future orientation with the possibility of upward social mobility
   b. results in less reliance on tradition
   c. results in the child's exposure to a number of adults who differ from one another but who all provide input as role models and teachers
   d. strongly influences adult relationships with children and produces changing philosophies of childrearing
   e. exerts a major force in providing continuity between generations; prepares children to carry out traditional social roles expected of adults in society

Section IV B

1.
   a. Hereditary factors - may be the result of an inherent lack of resistance to a disease organism, a trait that is an advantage in one environment but places the possessor at a disadvantage in another, or the consequence of intermarriage in a relatively narrow range of geographic, ethnic, or religious restrictions.
   b. Socioeconomic factors - such aspects of lower-class living conditions as crowding, poor sanitation, access to lead-containing substances, inadequate access to health services.

2.
   a. diet lacking in protein, vitamins, and iron leads to nutritional deficiency disorders and growth retardation in children.
   b. seek medical care only for serious or life-threatening illness, lack of preventive health care—no dental care, no prenatal care, no immunization.
   c. facilitates transfer of disease.

3. Nurses are products of their own cultural backgrounds, which influence their values, thoughts, and actions. When they are aware of their own culturally founded behavior, they are likely to be more sensitive to cultural behavior in others. They identify behaviors as characteristic of a culture rather than as "abnormal" and thus can relate more effectively with the families.

4.
   a. beliefs about diet and food practices.
   b. beliefs regarding birth, death, or other rituals.

5.
   a. establishing a resource file of pertinent information about the cultural and subcultural practices of people within the community.
   b. establishing a close relationship with families and other influential persons in the community.
   c. assessing his or her own attitudes and behaviors and those of other health workers toward people of varying cultures.

Section IV C

1. Lower-class — present orientation
   Middle-class — future orientation
2. Lower-class — Parents value the concrete and tangible rather than the abstract and are therefore less inclined to encourage these qualities in their children. Do not encourage education - no role models to support the value of education.
   Middle-class — Parents foster judgment, creativity, and resourcefulness in their children. Encourage and value education. Encourage children in activities that foster achievement.
3. Lower-class — Limited communication skills, such as simple grammar, inability to express abstractions, and ethnic dialects that hamper interactions with teachers from middle-class backgrounds.
   Middle-class — Parents are usually educated and foster reading and verbal skills. Children share the middle-class orientation of their teachers.

Chapter 4

Question   **Answer**

Section III

1.
   a. Family System Theory - The family is viewed as a system that continually inter-

acts with its members and the environment. The emphasis is on interaction.

  b. Developmental Theory - This theory uses a family life-cycle approach to compare the changing structure, function, and roles of the family at various stages of development, focusing on time as the central dimension. The theory delineates developmental tasks for the family much like the individual developmental tasks discussed in relation to personality development.

  c. Family Stress Theory - This theory explains how families react to stressful events and suggests factors that promote adaptation to these events.

2.
  a. caregiving
  b. nurturing
  c. training

3.
  a. 4
  b. 2
  c. 5
  d. 1
  e. 3

4. socialization

5.
  a. family size
  b. spacing of children
  c. ordinal position in family
  d. sibling interaction
  e. multiple births

6.
  a. T
  b. F
  c. F
  d. T

7.
  a. to promote the physical survival and health of the children
  b. to foster the skills and abilities necessary to be a self-sustaining adult
  c. to foster behavioral capabilities for maximizing cultural values and beliefs

8.
  a. parental age and previous experience
  b. father involvement
  c. effects of stress
  d. characteristics of the infant
  e. marital relationship

9.
  a. parents try to control their children's behavior and attitudes through rigid rules and regulations.

  b. parents allow children to regulate their own activity, viewing themselves as resources for the children, not role models.
  c. parents combine some practices from both the authoritarian and permissive styles, directing children's behavior and attitudes by emphasizing the reason for rules and negatively reinforcing deviations. Control is firm and consistent.

10.
  a. corporal punishment
  b. reasoning and scolding
  c. behavior modification
  d. consequences
  e. time out

11.
  a. 3
  b. 6
  c. 1
  d. 5
  e. 2
  f. 4

12. T

13.
  a. the task of telling the child that he is adopted.
  b. adolescents may use their adoption as a tool in defying parental authority or as a justification for aberrant behavior.

14.
  a. age and sex of the children
  b. the outcome of the divorce
  c. quality of parental care during the years following the divorce

15. at least half

16.
  a. Let relationships develop slowly and naturally.
  b. Don't criticize or belittle lost (or new) parents, or try to erase or replace them.
  c. Expect confused feelings, anxieties, competition for attention, and bids for loyalty.
  d. Communicate.
  e. Get help if needed.

Section IV A

1. Individuals with socially recognized statuses and positions who interact with one another on a regular, recurring basis in socially sanctioned ways.
2. events such as marriage, divorce, birth, death, abandonment, and incarceration.
3. Roles must be redefined or redistributed.
4.
  a. Nuclear — This family structure is highly adaptable, having the ability to adjust and reshape its structure when needed. It is free to move where there is opportunity and is

not dependent on the cooperative effort of other members. When there is wide geographic separation from the extended family, parents are faced with having no relatives readily available for advice, assistance and child care.

b. Single-parent — More liberal attitudes have made it possible to rear children without both parents being present in the home. Frequently children in these families are absorbed into the extended family.

c. Extended — More functional areas where land is the basis of wealth and sustenance. Here the family serves as the basic social, educational and productive unit, providing services and sharing resources. The needs of the individual are sublimated for the welfare of the family.

Section IV B

1. Altered self-image; need for realignment of role; feelings of anger, remorse, guilt, retaliation, and sorrow for oneself.

2. Parents tend to devote extra attention to the child because of feelings of guilt and lowered self-esteem. As a result, children often feel that the burden of the parent's happiness is on their shoulders.

3. Stress is both economic and emotional.
Fatigue and erratic parenting occur.
Loneliness is an additional problem.

4.
   a. age of child
   b. attitude of the father toward the wife's employment
   c. regularity with which the mother is away from home
   d. availability and quality of substitute child care

Section IV C

1.
   a. simple assumption that all normal people get married and have children.
   b. proof of biologic adequacy and demonstration of adulthood.
   c. fulfills a parent's wish for grandchildren and to perpetuate the family name and fortune.
   d. an attempt to save a tenuous marriage.

2.
   a. Integrate infants into the family unit
   Accommodate to new parenting and grandparenting roles
   Maintain the marital bond

b. Adolescents develop increasing autonomy
   Parents refocus on midlife marital and career issues
   Parents begin a shift toward concern for the older generation

3. Factors include cultural influences, social class, and economic resources.

Chapter 5

Question   Answer

Section III

1.
   a. 3
   b. 1
   c. 2
   d. 4
2.
   a. conception to birth
   b. birth to 28 days
   c. 1 month to 12 months
   d. 1 to 6 years
   e. 1 to 3 years
   f. 3 to 6 years
   g. 6 to 11 years
   h. 13 to 18 years
3.
   a. cephalocaudal, or head-to-tail
   b. proximodistal, or near-to-far
   c. mass to specific, or differentiation
4. sensitive periods
5.
   a. 2
   b. 1
   c. 4
   d. 3
6. physical growth
7. F
8. 110; 120; 40; 50
9.
   a. the difficult child
   b. the slow-to-warm-up child
   c. the easy child
10.
   a. oral stage - birth to 1 year
   b. anal stage - 1 to 3 years
   c. phallic stage - 3 to 6 years
   d. latency period - 6 to 12 years
   e. genital stage - 12 years and over
11.
   a. trust vs mistrust
   b. autonomy vs shame and doubt

    c. initiative vs guilt
    d. industry vs inferiority
    e. identity vs role confusion

12.
    a. 3, 5
    b. 1, 8
    c. 4, 7
    d. 2, 6

13.
    a. Preconventional morality
    b. Postconventional level
    c. Conventional level

14.
    a. 2
    b. 5
    c. 1
    d. 4
    e. 3

15. T

16. developmental retardation

17.
    a. sensorimotor development
    b. intellectual development
    c. socialization
    d. creativity
    e. self-awareness
    f. therapeutic value
    g. moral value

18. growth retardation

19. "an imbalance between environmental demands and a person's coping resources that...disrupts the equilibrium of the person"

20.
    a. increased verbally and physically aggressive behavior
    b. reduced persistence at problem solving
    c. greater sex-role stereotyping
    d. reduced creativity
    e. linked to obesity and high blood cholesterol levels
    f. implicit messages that promote alcohol consumption, smoking, violence, and promiscuous sexual activity

Section IV A

1. Although children vary in both their rate of growth and their acquisition of developmental skills, certain predictable patterns are universal and basic to all human beings.

2.
    a. 4
    b. 1, 2
    c. 2, 3
    d. 2
    e. 4, 5

3.
    a. trust vs mistrust (consistently meet the child's basic needs, provide loving care)
    b. autonomy vs shame and doubt (allow the child the opportunity to make choice)
    c. initiative vs guilt (encourage exploration of the environment; set realistic limits)
    d. industry vs inferiority (encourage competition and cooperation; assist in setting achievable goals)
    e. identity vs role confusion (provide positive feedback regarding appearance and activities)

4.
    a. no concept of right or wrong evident
    b. imitation of religious gestures and behaviors of others without comprehension of meaning
    c. imitation of religious behavior and following of parental religious beliefs as part of daily lives without real understanding of basic concepts
    d. strong interest in religion with acceptance of a deity; petitions to this deity made and expected to be answered
    e. realization that prayers are not always answered; initiation of modification or abandonment of religious practices; questioning of the religious standards of their parents

Section IV B

1. Infants with difficult or slow-to-warm-up patterns of behavior are more vulnerable to the development of behavioral problems in early and middle childhood. However, any child can develop behavior problems if there is dissonance between his or her temperament and the environment. When parents are unable to accept and deal with the child's behavior, there is a greater likelihood of subsequent behavioral problems.

2.
    a. even-tempered, regular and predictable habits, positive approach to new stimuli, adaptable to change
    b. highly active; irritable; irregular in habits; has negative withdrawal responses; slow to adapt to new routines, people, or situations
    c. inactive, moody, moderately irregular in functions, passively resistant to novelty or changes in routine, reacts negatively with mild intensity to new stimuli but adapts slowly with repeated contact

Section IV C

1.

    a. Provide a positive role model by developing television substitutes such as reading, athletics, physical conditioning, and hobbies.

    b. Construct a time chart of the child's activities.

    c. Discuss with the child what both believe to be a balanced set of activities.

    d. At the beginning of each week select appropriate programs from television schedules.

    e. Allow the child to select programs from this approved list.

    f. Limit child's viewing to two hours or less per day.

    g. Rule out TV at specific times.

    h. Make a list of alternate activities.

Chapter 6

Question   Answer

Section III

1.

    a. the appropriateness of the nurse's introduction to the child and family

    b. the nurse's explanation of her role in the health care setting and the purpose of the interview

    c. the inclusion of preliminary acquaintance conversation

    d. the nurse's assurance of privacy and confidentiality of the interview material

2.

    a. allows the nurse to obtain information concerning the health and developmental status of the child, factors that may influence the child's life, and cues to aspects in the child's health and development that may be a source of concern to the parents

    b. permits the nurse to allow for maximum freedom of expression while not allowing the interview to go off on tangents

    c. allows the nurse to make objective judgments concerning the perception of the parents, is useful in preventing the nurse's views from being interjected into the interview process, and aids in detecting cues from the parents that may aid in identifying problem areas

    d. allows the interviewee to sort out thoughts and feelings

    e. allows the nurse to see the problem from the parents' perspective

    f. facilitates the formulation of solutions because, in order for a problem to be solved, the nurse and parent must agree that one exists

    g. includes the parents in the problem-solving process and allows solutions to be proposed that will be adhered to by parents

    h. provides preventive methods so problems will not occur

    i. prevents the quality of the helping relationship from being altered

3.

    a. Long periods of silence

    b. Wide eyes and fixed facial expression

    c. Constant fidgeting or attempting to move away

    d. Nervous habits, e.g., tapping

    e. Sudden disruptions

    f. Looking around

    g. Yawning

    h. Frequently looking at a watch or clock

    i. Attempting to change topic of discussion

4.

    a. Learn proper terms of address.

    b. Use a positive tone of voice to convey interest

    c. Speak slowly and carefully, not loudly.

    d. Learn basic words and sentences of the family's language.

    e. Avoid professional jargon.

    f. Repeat important information more than once.

    g. Always give reason or purpose for a treatment.

    h. Use information written in the family's language.

    i. Offer the services of an interpreter.

    j. Learn from families and representatives of their culture methods of communicating information.

    k. Address intergenerational needs.

    l. Be sincere, open, and honest.

5.

    b

    a

    c

    d

6.   d

7.   writing; drawing; magic; play

8.   T

9.

    a. identifying information

    b. chief complaint

    c. present illness

    d. past history

    e. review of systems

f. family medical history
g. psychosocial history
h. sexual history
i. family history
j. nutritional assessment
10.
a. Family composition
b. Home and community environment
c. Occupation and education of family members
d. Cultural and religious traditions
11. sociogram
12. F
13. dietary intake; clinical examination; biochemical analysis
14. c

Section IV A

1. An appropriate introduction is crucial to establish a setting that is conducive to the interview process. The first component to this process is an introduction of the interviewer to the parents.
2. Some of the more common habits to communication are socializing, giving unrestricted advice, offering inappropriate reassurance, using stereotypic comments, using close-ended questions, interrupting the client, talking more than the interviewee, and deliberately changing the focus.
3. A number of techniques are effective. These include third-person technique; storytelling; using books, "what if" questions, three wishes, rating games, word association games, sentence completion, drawing, magic, and playing.
4. It is important to include the parent in the problem-solving process because a parent who is included will be more likely to follow through on a course of action. In addition, a parent may have already tried a particular solution. Encouraging participation may prevent the nurse from suggesting a solution that the patient has already tried.

Section IV B

1.
a. Learn proper terms of address.
b. Use a positive tone of voice to convey interest.
c. Speak slowly and carefully, not loudly.
d. Learn basic words and sentences of the family's language.
e. Avoid professional jargon.
f. Repeat important information more than once.
g. Always give reason or purpose for a treatment.
h. Use information written in the family's language.
i. Offer the services of an interpreter.
j. Learn from families and representatives of their culture methods of communicating information.
k. Address intergenerational needs.
l. Be sincere, open, and honest.
2. The nurse can redirect the focus of the interview by saying that they can talk about the other children later in the interview.
3. Since Susan has been in this country only 6 months, she may have not received her immunization. It is extremely important for the nurse to obtain an accurate record of immunizations from Mrs. Fernandez.
4. The nurse should obtain information concerning the state of health, age, and presence of illness of first-degree relatives.
5.
a. Home (Home observation for management of the environment)
b. HSQ (Home Screening Questionnaire)

Section IV C

1. A dietary history should include information regarding the family mealtime, preparation of food, pattern of eating and of meals, likes and dislikes of the child, appetite, allergies, feeding problems, family history of illnesses, pattern of weight gain, the child's pattern of exercise, and the amount of money spent on food.
2. The three methods include 24-hour recall, food diary, and food frequency record.
3. Anthropometry is the measurement of height, weight, head circumference, proportions, skinfold thickness and arm circumference. Skinfold thickness is a measurement of the body's fat content and would be useful in determining whether Gwen is obese.
4. Gwen should be told what is being done and why. She should be told that various measurements such as height, weight, and skinfold thickness will be taken to determine how big and tall she has become. If blood is to be drawn, she should be told why.
5.
a. Altered nutrition: more than body requirements related to eating practices
b. Altered nutrition: more than body requirements related to knowledge deficit of parents

Chapter 7

Question   Answer

Section III

1.
   a. minimizing the stress and anxiety associated with body part assessment
   b. fostering a trusting nurse-child-parent relationship
   c. allowing for maximum preparation of the child
   d. preserving the essential security of the parent-child relationship
   e. maximizing the accuracy and reliability of the assessment findings

2.
   a. Assess child for reason for uncooperative behavior.
   b. Try to involve child and parent in process.
   c. Avoid prolonged explanations about examining procedure.
   d. Use a firm, direct approach regarding expected behavior.
   e. Perform examination as quickly as possible.
   f. Have attendant gently restrain child.
   g. Minimize any disruptions or stimulation.

3.
   a. growth measurements
   b. physiologic measurements
   c. general appearance
   d. skin
   e. lymph nodes
   f. head and neck
   g. eyes
   h. ears
   i. nose
   j. mouth and throat
   k. chest
   l. lungs
   m. heart
   n. abdomen
   o. genitalia
   p. anus
   q. back and extremities
   r. neurologic assessment
   s. developmental assessment

4. d
5. respiration, pulse, and temperature
6. for a full minute
7. b

8.
   b
   c
   d
   a
9. When assessing the head of an 8-month-old, the nurse should record the general shape, symmetry, presence of patent sutures, fontanels, fractures and swelling, and the condition of the scalp.
10. d
11. F
12. primitive
13. F
14. birth through 6 years
15. T
16. Differs in items included in the test, the test form, and the interpretation.

Section IV A

1. You should observe Tia for signs of readiness such as her willingness to talk to you, make eye contact, accept the offered equipment, allow physical contact, or choose to sit on the examining table. Several methods might be used to facilitate the exam process. You could tell a story or use a puppet. Since Tia needs to have a developmental assessment, you might want to begin with this aspect of the exam because it might be perceived by Tia as a game.
2. Tia is 3 years of age, so she can have her height taken while standing. She should be encouraged to stand as tall and straight as possible.
3. Additional assessment information might include Tia's parents' patterns of growth, whether her growth pattern has been steady, and her nutritional intake. In addition, you might want to employ growth charts standardized for Asian populations to see if her height and weight are normal for this group.
4. Tia may not understand that she should not bite down on the thermometer or that she has to keep the thermometer under her tongue and her mouth closed.
5. Tia should have a complete vision assessment that includes binocularity and acuity. To test for binocularity, you might use the corneal light reflex test or the cover test. To test for acuity, you might use the Blackbird Preschool Vision Screening System.

Section IV B

1. After the general appearance section the skin is assessed.
2. The infant's height is obtained in the recumbent position by fully extending the child's body. The school-age child's height is obtained by having the child stand straight. Height should be recorded to the nearest 1/8 in. or 1 mm.
3. Radial pulses can be obtained if the child is over 2 years of age. The infant's pulse should be taken apically, and the school-age child's can be taken radially.
4. Information in this area includes the child's personality, level of activity, reaction of stress, requests frustration; interaction with others, degree of alertness, and response to stimuli.
5. use a Crib-o-gram or tympanometry
6. quality, intensity, rate, and rhythm
7. Instruct the child to hold his breath; this causes the heart rate to remain steady.

Section IV C

1. The parent is told that the purpose of the test is to help the nurse observe what the child can do at this age and that the results of the performance will be explained after all items have been completed. It should be emphasized that this is not an intelligence test.
2. The parent is asked whether the child's performance is typical of his behavior at other times.
3. The method employed is a failure to perform an item that is passed by 90% of children the child's age or any item that falls completely to the left of the age line.
4. Items are scored as follows: P, passing; F, failing; and R, refusal.
5. All children with questionable or abnormal results should be rescreened before a referral for further diagnostic testing is made.

Chapter 8

Question   Answer

Section III

1. the entrance of air into the upper airway replacing the lung fluid, initiation of breathing, and a lowering of the surface tension in the alveoli
2. F
3. a

4.
   a. large surface area
   b. thin layer of subcutaneous fat
   c. inability to shiver
5. d
6. T
7. heart rate, respiratory effort, muscle tone, color and reflex irritability
8. 10
9. 6 to 8
10. an alert and active infant, active gag reflex, increased heart and respiratory rate, increased gastric and respiratory secretions, and passage of meconium
11. F
12. F
13. T
14. b
15. posture, behavior, skin, head, eyes, ears, nose, mouth, and throat, neck, chest, lungs, heart, abdomen, genitalia, back and anus extremities, and neurologic system
16. two arteries
17.
   a. maintenance of patent airway
   b. maintenance of stable body temperature
   c. protection from injury and infection
   d. provision of optimum nutrition
   e. promotion of parent-infant attachment
   f. preparation for discharge and home care
18. T
19. the pH of the skin surface, which is slightly acidic.
20. b
21. T
22. postpartum hospitalizations are shorter, and more deliveries are being performed at home.
23. breast-feeding, maternal fatigue and depression, bonding, neonatal jaundice, and excessive infant crying

Section IV A

1. heart, respiratory effort, muscle tone, reflex irritability, and color
2. below 100 beats/min
3. 7 to 10
4. The behaviors that are observed include an initial period of alertness, vigorous suck, initially elevated heart and respiratory rates, active bowel sounds, and falling temperature
5. c

Section IV B

1. perinatal mortality and morbidity are related to gestational age and weight
2. 30 and 42 hours of age
3. posture, square window, arm recoil, popliteal angle, scarf sign, and heel-to-ear maneuver
4. his weight falls between the 10th and 90th percentile

Section IV C

1. 33 and 35.5 cm (12 to 13 inches); microcephaly or craniostenosis should be suspected.
2. The areas to assess include observing the lids for edema, symmetry of the eyes, presence of tears, presence of discharge, presence of corneal reflex, presence of pupillary reflex, presence of nystagmus or strabismus, and color of the iris.
3. The infant is able to respond to his environment by moving his head and/or limbs and staring at objects in the environment such as a mobile or a face.

Section IV D

1.
   a. Ineffective airway clearance related to excess mucus, improper positioning
   b. Potential altered body temperature related to immature temperature control, change in environmental temperature
   c. Potential for infection related to deficient immunologic defenses, environmental factors
   d. Potential for trauma related to physical helplessness
   e. Altered nutrition: less than body requirements (potential) related to immaturity, parental knowledge deficit.
   f. Altered family processes related to maturational crisis, birth of term infant, change in family unit
2.
   a. position on right side or abdomen after feeding
   b. keep diapers, clothing, and blankets loose
   c. clean nares of crusted material
   d. check for patency of nares
3. The reason that clothes are kept loose is that infants are abdominal breathers; this intervention allows for maximal expansion of the lungs.
4. The infant is in the first stage of reactivity. During this time he is alert and awake and can establish eye-to-eye contact with the parents, facilitating the development of attachment.
5. Criteria include breathing that is regular and unlabored, normal respiratory rate, and gastric aspirates of 20 ml or less.

6. The parents should be instructed in routine baby care such as feeding, bathing, and umbilical and circumcision care.
   They should also be encouraged to participate in parenting classes, and the use of care restraints should be discussed.

Section IV E

1. Specific behaviors that might be assessed include the following: the parent reaching out for the baby when she is brought into the room, referring to the infant by name, talking about who the child looks like, speaking about the uniqueness of the infant, the type of body contact used, types of stimulation, and whether or not the parents avoid eye contact.
2. This is important because the ability to parent is largely dependent on the type of parenting the parents received as children, as this may influence the attachment process.
3. Altered parenting related to knowledge deficit or lack of available role models
4.
   a. allow parents to see and hold the infant as soon as possible.
   b. Perform eye care after the parents have met the infant.
   c. Identify the infant's unique behaviors.
   d. Observe and assess the reciprocity of cues between infant and parents.
   e. Assess variables affecting the attachment process.
   f. Observe for behaviors indicating attachment.

Chapter 9

Question   Answer

Section III

1. presenting part; maternal pelvis
2. a
3. clavicle
4. facial nerve paralysis
5. proper positioning
6.
   a. C
   b. I
   c. I
   d. C
   e. C
   f. I

7.
   a. size
   b. gestational age
   c. mortality
8. Determine presence of abdominal distention; determine any signs of regurgitation, residual, or emesis. Assess stools and bowel sounds.
9. higher
10. c
11. acid mantle of the skin
12. 1, 3, 2
13. hyperbilirubinemia
14. jaundice
15. This occurs because of the immaturity of hepatic function combined with increased hemolysis of excess red blood cells.
16. phototherapy
17. c
18. T
19. meningitis, and shock
20. abdominal distention, blood in stools, gastric retention, localized abdominal wall erythema
21. d
22. phenobarbital, chlorpromazine, diazepam, or paregoric
23. Lyme disease
24. T
25. phenylalanine hydroxylase
26. screening with the Guthrie test
27. F

Section IV A

1.
   a. a vaguely outlined area of edematous tissue situated over the portion of the scalp that presents in a vertex delivery. The swelling consists of serum, blood, or both, accumulated in the tissues above the bone, and it may extend beyond the bone margins. It is present at or shortly after birth.
   b. formed when blood vessels rupture during labor or delivery to produce bleeding into the area between the bone and its periosteum. The boundaries are sharply demarcated and do not extend beyond the limits of the bone. Swelling is usually minimum at birth and increases on the second or third day.

2.
   a. detection of complications, such as subdural hematoma, infection, or intraventricular hemorrhage
   b. parental support

Section IV B

1. The most meaningful method of classification is one that encompasses all three methods, i.e., size, gestational age, and mortality
2.
   a. placing infant in a humidified Isolette or radiant warmer
   b. monitoring temperature hourly
   c. avoiding situations that predispose to chilling
3. High-risk infants have deficient immunologic defenses and are also exposed to many sources of nosocomial infections.
4. Altered nutrition: less than body requirements related to inability to ingest nutrients because of immaturity or illness.
5. The infant should be weighed daily and should exhibit a steady weight gain.
6. Assessment of the skin reveals that the skin remains clean and intact with no evidence of irritation or injury
7.
   a. keep parents informed of infant's progress
   b. facilitate parent-infant attachment
   c. facilitate sibling-infant attachment
   d. prepare for discharge
8. Since the infant is in an ICU, the parents may not have had time to become acquainted with and attached to their infant. Encouraging visitation counteracts interruptions of the bonding process.

Section IV C

1.
   a. immaturity of hepatic functions
   b. increased bilirubin load from increased hemolysis of red blood cells
2.
   a. after 24 hours
   b. by the third day
   c. from the fifth to the seventh day
3.
   a. Shield the infant's eyes with an opaque mask.
   b. Place the infant nude under the fluorescent light.
   c. Monitor body temperature.
   d. Give 25% additional fluid volume.

Section IV D

1. cross-contamination. The sources of this could include humidifying apparatus, suction machines, indwelling catheters, poor handwashing and inadequate housecleaning.

2. Some of the signs of sepsis are poor temperature control, pallor, hypotension, edema, respiratory distress, diminished or increased activity, full fontanel, poor feeding, vomiting, diarrhea, jaundice, and an infant not doing well.
3. recognition of the existing problem.

Section IV E

1. Michael experienced severe asphyxia at birth.
2. early recognition
3. monitoring the abdomen for distention, observing bilious vomitus, and occult or frank blood in stool.

Section IV F

1. It occurs as a result of the hyperplasia and hypertrophy of the islet cells in utero. The islet cells continue to excrete large amounts of insulin after birth, resulting in decreased blood glucose levels.
2. Feeding is begun early to prevent hypoglycemia.
3. hypoglycemia, central nervous system signs, polycythemia, hyperbilirubinemia, sepsis, and respiratory distress syndrome.

Chapter 10

Question   Answer

Section III

1. doubled
2. 4 months
3. d
4.
   a. greater proportion of extracellular fluid
   b. immaturity of renal structures
5. b
6. a
7. T
8. c
9.
   a. the ability to discriminate the mother from other individuals
   b. the achievement of object permanence
10. T
11. preference for mother demonstrated by behaviors such as clinging to the parent, crying, and turning away from the stranger.
12. a
13. developmental
14. mirrors, bright toys to hold, rattles or bells, soft squeeze toys, mobiles, and swings.

15. Parents should be aware that this child will have to be watched more closely, and that extra precautions regarding safety will need to be taken. This child benefits from increased opportunity for gross motor activities.
16. F
17. age of child-6 = number of teeth
18. protection
19. fluoride: .25 mg
20. F
21.
    a. the digestive tract is not able to digest them
    b. food allergies may develop
    c. the extrusion reflex is still strong
    d. inability to push food away
22. infant cereal; iron
23. T
24. a
25. F
26. c
27. local tenderness, erythema, and swelling at the injection site and a low-grade fever
28. c
29. asphyxiation by foreign material
30. d

Section IV A

1. Yes. Jerry should have at least doubled his birth weight by at least 5 months. The average infant gains at least 1.5 pounds a month until 5 months old.
2. Jerry's developmental milestones are assessed as follows: when supine lifts head off table, sits erect momentarily, bears full weight on feet, transfers objects from hand to hand, rakes at a small object, bangs cube on table, produces vowel sounds and chained syllables, vocalizes four distinct vowel sounds, plays peekaboo, fears strangers when mother disappears, and imitates simple acts.
3. You should stress to Mrs. Backer that this behavior is normal and indicates good parental attachment. Mrs. Backer should be encouraged to allow clingy behavior and to encourage close friends or relatives to visit often.
4.
   a. frozen teething ring to chew on
   b. topical analgesics such as Baby Ora-Jel
5. Jerry's lack of interest in breast-feeding may indicate his desire to be weaned. You should suggest that Jerry might be weaned to a cup, that it should be done gradually by replacing one feeding at time, with the nighttime feeding the last to be replaced, and not allowing the child to take a bottle to bed.

6.

   a. give fluoride supplements if the water supply is deficit

   b. clean teeth with a damp cloth

   c. do not include concentrated sugars in the diet

   d. do not coat pacifiers with honey

   e. never allow a bottle to be taken to bed or during a nap

Section IV B

1. Behaviors include searching for objects that have fallen, imitating sounds, showing great interest in mirror image.

2.

   a. the reason for the concern

   b. the frequency and duration of waking

   c. the usual bedtime routine

   d. the number of night-time feedings

   e. the interventions Rachel's mother attempted

3.

   a. Rachel should be started on cereal first

   b. cereal should be mixed with formula

   c. spoon feeding should be first introduced after the infant has had some formula

   d. the infant will at first push spoon away but be persistent

   e. introduce new foods one at a time. New foods are fed in small amounts (about 1 tsp) and for a period of 4 to 7 days

   f. as the amount of solids increases, she should decrease the amount of formula

   g. Do not introduce foods by mixing them with formula in bottle

Section IV C

1. Live virus vaccines should not be given to infants with a febrile illness, acquired passive immunity, a known allergic response to a previously administered vaccine or substance in the vaccine, or who have immunodeficiency diseases or who have received immunosuppressive therapy or who have a sibling at home receiving such therapy.

2.

   a. proper storage such as refrigeration and exposure to light

   b. DPT vaccines should always be administered intramuscularly with a needle of adequate length to deposit the antigen deep in the muscle mass. Care should be taken to prevent tracking of fluid into the skin.

3. The safest site for the administration of immunizations is the vastus lateralis or ventrogluteal

4.

   a. inquire about reactions to previously administered DPT vaccines

   b. advise parents of side effects such as fever, soreness, redness and swelling at site, malaise

   c. recommend the use of acetaminophen if fever occurs

   d. advise parents to notify the physician if any unusual symptoms such as loss of consciousness, convulsions, high fever, or systemic allergic reaction occur

Section IV D

1. Such developmental landmarks include crawling, standing, cruising, walking, climbing, pulling on objects, throwing objects, picking up small objects, exploring by mouthing, exploring away from parent

2.

   a. place guard around heating appliances, fireplace, or furnace

   b. keep electrical wires hidden

   c. keep hanging tablecloth out of reach

   d. apply a sunscreen when infant is exposed to sunlight

   e. place plastic guards over electrical outlets, place furniture in front of outlets

3. The infant is now mobile and could drown in a tub if allowed to get in the bathroom

4. Infants at this age still explore objects by mouthing them and might choke on a small object.

5. The child may think the medication is candy and eat some and might accidentally be poisoned.

6. You should suggest that the grandparents' homes be accident-proofed as well.

Chapter 11

Question   **Answer**

Section III

1. T

2. injudicious use of vitamin supplements

3. b

4. F

5. loss of appetite, diminished taste sensation, delayed healing, skin lesions, alopecia, diarrhea, growth failure, and retarded sexual maturity.

6. liver, red meat, poultry, shellfish, green leafy vegetables, dried fruits, nuts, enriched cereals and breads, potatoes, molasses, and infant formula.

7. less than 2, 2 years, 30%, 40%

8. d

9. from the findings of the history

10. Lactase

11. diarrhea, abdominal pain, distention, flatus after ingesting milk

12.
    c
    d
    a
    b

13.
   a. diet of the breast-feeding mother
   b. time of day when attacks occur
   c. relationship of the attack to feeding time
   d. presence of specific family members during attacks and habits such as smoking
   e. activity of caregiver before, during, and after the crying
   f. characteristics of the cry
   g. measures used to relieve the crying and their effectiveness

14. T

15. to terminate the ruminating behavior and restore normal feeding patterns

16. F

17. socially isolated, have inadequate support systems, had poor parenting as a child

18. is the provision of adequate nutrition for growth

19.
   a. provide a quiet, unstimulating environment
   b. maintain a calm, even temperament
   c. talk to child by giving directions about eating
   d. follow child's rhythm of feeding
   e. develop a structured routine
   f. be persistent
   g. maintain a face-to-face posture with the child

20.
   a. Infants with one or more severe ALTEs requiring CPR or vigorous stimulation
   b. Preterm infants who continue to have apnea at time of discharge
   c. Siblings of 2 or more SIDS victims
   d. Infants with certain types of diseases or conditions such as central hypoventilation

21. the usual sequence of events that occur after the infant is found

22. to avoid any suggestions of responsibility on the part of the parents

23. cardiopneumogram

24. home monitoring, methylxanthines

25.
   a. removal of leads from infant when not attached to monitor
   b. unplugging power cord from electrical outlet when not plugged into monitor
   c. using safety covers on electrical outlets

26. c

Section IV A

1. The nurse should have assessed the cultural food preferences of the Bacons. Seventh Day Adventists are often vegetarians. They may also have a lack of knowledge of how to meet their child's nutritional needs on this type of diet.

2. exactly what the diet includes and excludes

3.
   a. teaching the Bacons to include grains, beans, milk products (if allowed) to meet protein and niacin requirements
   b. teaching the Bacons to include enriched cereals
   c. teaching the Bacons to include juices containing vitamin C
   d. suggesting that they use soy-based formulas
   e. suggesting that they use a variety of foods in the diet
   f. teaching them about the safety and digestibility of solid food

4. If the interventions were successful, the infant would begin to gain weight; the infant would not exhibit signs of niacin deficiency such as stomatitis, scaly dermatitis, diarrhea, or lethargy; and the parents would be able to verbalize and provide a nutritionally adequate diet for the child.

Section IV B

1.
   a. identify mothers and fathers at risk
   b. recognize characteristics of parents
   c. identify children who fail to thrive

2. Some of the characteristics would include: (1) growth failure; (2) developmental retardation; (3) apathy; (4) poor hygiene; (5) withdrawal behavior; (6) feeding or eating disorders, such as rumination; (7) avoidance of eye-to-eye contact; (8) no fear of strangers; and (9) minimum smiling

3. the child gains a minimum of 1 to 2 oz a day and whether the infant responds positively to feeding practices

4. Altered parenting related to poverty, neglect or lack of knowledge.

Section IV C

1.
   a. inform the parents that the child probably died from SIDS
   b. ask as few questions as possible
   c. avoid giving any indication of guilt
2. to allow them an opportunity for a last visit with the child
3.
   a. make home visits as soon as possible
   b. provide literature about SIDS
   c. refer parents to local foundation

Section IV D

1. educating the parents regarding the equipment, observing the infant's status, and immediately intervening during apneic periods
2. Monitors can cause electrical burns and electrocution.
3. The utility company is informed because, if there is a power outage, some provision of emergency power may be provided. The rescue squad is notified because in the event that the infant stops breathing, they will be aware of the problem, and help may arrive more quickly.
4. encouraging other family members to become familiar with the equipment, read and interpret signals, administer CPR, and stay with infant
5. Vomiting usually refers to the forcible ejection of stomach contents. Spitting up refers to the dribbling of unswallowed formula from the infant's mouth immediately after feedings.

Section IV E

1. are retarded
2. increasing social awareness, teaching verbal skills, and decreasing unacceptable behavior

Chapter 12

Question   Answer

Section III

1. 12 months; 3 years of age
2. 2 1/2
3. T
4. Because the abdominal musculature is not yet well developed and because the legs, though elongating, are still short in relation to the rest of the body.

5. 20/20; 20/40
6. elimination
7. locomotion
8.
   a. differentiation of self from others, particularly the mother
   b. toleration of separation from the parent
   c. ability to withstand delayed gratification
   d. control over bodily functions
   e. acquisition of socially acceptable behavior
   f. verbal means of communication
   g. ability to interact with others in a less ego-centric manner
9. autonomy; doubt; shame
10.
   a. negativism
   b. ritualism
11. tolerate delayed gratification
12. e
13. preconceptual phase
14. a
15.
   a. 2
   b. 3
   c. 1
   d. 5
   e. 4
16. T
17
   a. the child's emergence from a symbiotic fusion with the mother
   b. those achievements that mark children's assumption of their own individual characteristics in the environment
18. F
19. 300; 65
20. independence
21. d
22. parallel
23. 15 months
24. latter half of the second year
25. T
26. firstborn
27. F
28. time out
29. independence
30. the opportunities of a "no" answer
31. physiologic anorexia
32. 1 Tbsp
33. 2 1/2
34. brushing; flossing
35. fluoride, reduced
36. d
37. Injuries
38. There is a need to emphasize safety awareness in parents.

39. The rule of fours is a guide to determining when a child has outgrown a special car restraint system. According to this rule, a child should use this restraint until he weighs about 40 pounds, or is 40 inches tall; then a regular car restraint system can be used.

40. scald burns

41. improper storage of toxic agents

Section IV A

1.
   a. slightly below the 75th percentile
   b. falls at the 75th percentile

2. Growth slows considerably during the toddler years. A toddler gains approximately 4 to 6 pounds and grows 3 inches per year. Growth occurs in spurts and plateaus during toddlerhood.

3.
   a. goes up and down stairs alone, using both feet on each step; picks up objects without falling; and can kick a ball forward without overbalancing
   b. can build a tower of 6 to 7 cubes; turns the pages of a book one at a time; can imitate vertical and circular strokes when drawing; and turns knob
   c. uses two- to three-word phrases; uses the pronouns I, me, and you; and talks incessantly

4. This is characteristic of parallel play, which is typical during the toddler years.

5.
   a. toys should be purchased using safety and developmental level as guidelines
   b. child should be allowed to choose the toys he wishes to play with at a given time
   c. child should be allowed unrestricted motor activity within safe limits

6. b

7.
   a. if drinking water is not fluoridated, provide fluoride supplements
   b. arrange a visit to the dentist so the child may become familiar with the equipment
   c. introduce the use of a soft toothbrush as part of the child's bedtime regimen
   d. encourage the consumption of a low-cariogenic diet

Section IV B

1. By their persistent "no" response to every request.

2. negative response

3. As an assertion of self-control and an attempt to control the environment, it increases independence.

4. Toddlers assert their independence by violently objecting in this manner to restrictions on their behavior.

5. Because the growth rate slows, there is a decrease in nutritional needs

6.
   a. unpredictable table manners
   b. rituals involving mealtime and utensils
   c. inability to sit through family mealtimes
   d. food fads or jags

7. Because the eating habits established in the first 2 or 3 years of life tend to have lasting effects

8. Fears of separation

9.
   a. Bedtime rituals are helpful
   b. Use of transitional objects

Section IV C

1.
   a. child protection
   b. parent education

2. The toddler is unrestricted because of increased locomotion and is unaware of danger in the environment.

3.
   a. motor vehicle injuries
   b. drowning
   c. burns
   d. poisoning
   e. falls
   f. aspiration and suffocation
   g. bodily damage

4.
   a. matches and cigarette lighters
   b. sources of water—tubs, swimming pools
   c. medications, toxic agents, plants
   d. unguarded stairways
   e. tools, garden equipment, and firearms

5.
   a. d, g, i
   b. a, e, f
   c. c, h
   d. b, d, e

6. Approved restraints properly installed and applied can reduce fatalities and injuries.

Chapter 13

Question   Answer

Section III

1. 3; fifth
2. slow; stabilize
3.
   a. how to interact and relate to other children and adults
   b. appropriate sex role functions and socially acceptable behavior
   c. right and wrong and the types of reward or punishment associated with each
4. initiative
5. superego; conscience
6. readiness, scholastic learning
7.
   a. the preconceptual phase (ages 2 to 4)
   b. the phase of intuitive thought (ages 4 to 7)
8. There is a shift from totally egocentric thought to social awareness and ability to consider other viewpoints.
9. language, speech, egocentric
10. causality
11. magical
12. T
13.
   a. They can relate to unfamiliar people easily.
   b. They tolerate brief separations from parents with little or no protest.
14. T
15. Telegraphic
16. 2100
17.
   a. The preschooler is able to verbalize his request for independence
   b. The preschooler can perform many tasks independently
18. associative
19. 2 1/2, 3
20.
   a. they become friends for the child in times of loneliness
   b. they accomplish what the child is still attempting
   c. they experience what the child wants to forget or remember
21. a
22.
   a. learning group cooperation
   b. adjusting to various sociocultural differences
   c. coping with frustration, dissatisfaction, and anger

23.
   a. whether the facility is licensed
   b. qualifications of the staff
   c. student-to-staff ratio
   d. discipline policy
   e. environmental safety precautions
   f. provision of meals
   g. sanitary conditions
   h. adequate indoor and outdoor space per child
   i. fee schedule
   j. health practices of agency
24. personal observation
25.
   a. determine what the child thinks
   b. be honest with responses
26. Masturbation
27. 2; 4
28. The child is using his rapidly growing vocabulary to interact with the environment. However, the rate of vocabulary acquisition does not parallel the child's advancing mental ability or degree of comprehension.
29.
   a. fear of the dark
   b. fear of being left alone
   c. fear of animals
   d. fear of ghosts
   e. fear of sexual matters
   f. fear of objects or persons associated with pain
30. Actively involve them in finding practical methods to deal with frightening experiences.
31. DASE
32. toddlers; Four; 5
33. The quality of the food consumed is more important than the quantity.
34.
   a. they have difficulty going to sleep after daytime activity and stimulation
   b. they develop bedtime fears
   c. they awaken during the night
   d. they have nightmares or sleep terrors
   e. they prolong going to sleep through elaborate rituals
35.
   a. to preserve the deciduous teeth
   b. to teach good dental habits
36. T

Section IV A

1.
   a. slightly above the 25th percentile
   b. falls at the 25th percentile
2. Physical growth slows and stabilizes during this time. The average weight gain is about 5 lb. (2.3

kg) per year, and height increases by about 2.5 to 3 in. (6.75 to 7.5 cm) per year.

3.

   a. skips and hops on alternate feet; throws and catches ball well; and walks backward with heel to toe

   b. ties shoelaces; uses scissors well; and prints a few letters, numbers, or words

   c. has a vocabulary of 2100 words; uses 6- to 8-word sentences; and names four or more colors

4. The functions served by these playmates are accomplished as the child gets older. Most children give up these friends when the group process becomes more important, usually when they enter school.

5.

   a. balls, shovels, ladders, swings, slides, sleds, wagons, blocks

   b. blocks, cars, sandboxes, old adult clothes

   c. paper, crayons, finger paints, chalk, paste, musical toys

   d. books, puzzles, records, table games

6. Because of improved gross motor skills and increasing independence, the preschooler is susceptible to injuries from such activities as playing in the street, riding a tricycle, chasing after balls, or forgetting safety regulations when crossing streets.

Section IV B

1. The social climate, type of guidance, and attitude toward the children that is fostered by the teacher or leader rather than whether or not structured learning is imposed.

2.

   a. licensing of the facility

   b. the center's daily program

   c. teacher qualifications

   d. child-to-staff ratio

   e. environmental safety

   f. sanitary conditions

   g. provision of meals

   h. indoor and outdoor space per child; discipline policy

   i. fee schedule

3.

   a. meet the director

   b. meet some of the caregivers or teachers

   c. systematically evaluate the facility in comparison with others

   d. observe the program in action

4.

   a. present the idea of school as exciting and pleasurable

   b. talk to the child about the activities that he will participate in at school

   c. provide the school with detailed information about the child's home environment, such as familiar routines, food preferences, etc.

   d. introduce the child to the teacher and familiarize him with the school

Section IV C

1. At about age 3 years, children are aware of anatomic differences between the sexes and are concerned with how the anatomy of the opposite sex works. They are really concerned about eliminative functions. This leads to physical exploration and questions to obtain more information.

2.

   a. giving no answer

   b. giving too much information

3.

   a. this allows parents to identify the child's beliefs, and enables them to reinforce or correct the information

   b. this avoids the establishment of a double standard in which the child receives conflicting information

4. Inability to fall asleep, bedtime fears, waking during the night, nightmares, prolonging bedtime through rituals.

5.

   a. ignore attention-seeking behavior

   b. establish and consistently apply a reasonable bedtime ritual

   c. alleviate sources of fear by keeping a light on, providing a favorite toy, etc.

   d. decrease levels of stimuli before bedtime

6. The decreased quantity of food that the preschooler consumes.

7. Advise parents to keep a weekly record of the child's diet in order to accurately estimate the intake of food at each meal. This should be evaluated at the end of a week's time. In most instances, the child has consumed more than the parent realizes.

Chapter 14

Question   **Answer**

Section III

1.

   a. recent exposure to a known case

    b. history of prodromal symptoms or evidence of constitutional symptoms
    c. history of previous immunizations
    d. previous history of having the disease

2.
    a. prevent spread of infection to others
    b. prevent complications
    c. provide comfort measures
    d. support the child and family

3. immunization

4.
    a. prevention of the disease
    b. control the spread of the disease to others

5.
    a. those undergoing steroid or other immunosuppressive therapy
    b. those who have a generalized malignancy
    c. those who have an immunologic disorder

6.
    a. cool baths
    b. use of lotions such as calamine
    c. avoid overheating
    d. keep nails short and smooth
    e. administer an antipruritic medication

7. Inflammation of the conjunctiva

8.
    a. obstruction of the nasolacrimal duct
    b. bacterial infection

9. purulent drainage

10. T

11. F

12. b

13.
    a. keeping the eye clean
    b. properly administering ophthalmic medication

14. prevention of infection in other family members

15.
    a. aphthous stomatitis
    b. herpetic stomatitis

16.
    a. 1
    b. 2
    c. 1
    d. 2
    e. 2

17. Intestinal parasitic diseases

18.
    a. their hand-to-mouth activity
    b. their uncontrolled evacuation habits

19.
    a. identification of the organism
    b. treatment of the infection
    c. prevention of initial infection or reinfection

20. preventive education of children and families regarding good hygiene and health habits

21. Giardiasis

22. Enterobiasis; pinworm

23. T

24.
    a. general irritability
    b. restlessness
    c. poor sleep
    d. bedwetting
    e. distractibility
    f. short attention span

25. tape test

26. It provides that certain potentially hazardous drugs and household products be sold in child-resistant containers.

27.
    a. infants and toddlers explore their environment through oral experimentation
    b. the sense of taste is less discriminating in small children, and many unpalatable substances are ingested
    c. toddlers and preschoolers are developing autonomy and initiative, which increases their curiosity and exploration
    d. imitation is a powerful motivator, especially when combined with a lack of awareness of danger

28.
    a. assessment
    b. gastric decontamination
    c. family support
    d. prevention of recurrence

29. ipecac syrup

30.
    a. used in young infants in whom ipecac is contraindicated
    b. used if the patient is comatose or convulsing or requires a protected airway
    c. used if the ingested poison is rapidly absorbed

31. F

32. aspiration

33. T

34. F

35. Acetaminophen; hepatic

36. emesis; lavage, N-acetylcysteine (Mucomyst)

37. twice

38. nervous

39. F

40.
    a. calcium disodium edetate (EDTA)
    b. dimercaprol (BAL)
    c. penicillamine
    d. succimer (chemet)

41. Child maltreatment

42. T

43.
    a. parental characteristics

b. characteristics of the child
c. environmental characteristics

44. c
45. d
46.
  a. protect the child from further abuse
  b. support the child and family
  c. prevent abuse

47.
  a. incest
  b. molestation
  c. exhibitionism
  d. child pornography
  e. child prostitution
  f. pedophilia

Section IV A

1. Through a tape test or inspection of the anal area while the child sleeps
2.
  a. identify the parasite
  b. eradicate the organism
  c. prevent reinfection

Section IV B

1.
  a. obtain vital signs and initiate any needed respiratory and/or circulatory support; institute measures to reduce effects of shock; anticipate and prepare for potential problems
  b. induce vomiting if indicated; administer antidotes; assist with gastric lavage; be aware of indications and contraindications for the various decontamination procedures
  c. unaccusingly explore the circumstances of the accident; avoid premature attempts at education regarding prevention of recurrence; remain calm and support child and parent; avoid admonishing for negligence
  d. discussion difficulties of constantly safeguarding young children; make a follow-up home visit for assessment of potential hazards; ask specific questions to isolate risk factors; emphasize proper storage

2.
  a. S
  b. A
  c. S
  d. S
  e. A

3.
  a. "If you suspected that your child ingested a poison, what would you do first?"
  b. "Do you have ipecac syrup in your home?"
  c. "Should you always make the child vomit following the ingestion of poison?"
  d. "If you suspected that your child had taken a poison, but there was no signs of illness and the child denied doing so, what would you do?"

Section IV C

1.
  a. old housing
  b. presence of a lead smelter nearby
  c. use of folk remedies
  d. contaminated water in formula
  e. heavy automobile exhaust

2.
  a. hyperactivity, aggression, impulsiveness, decreased interest in play, lethargy, irritability, hearing impairment, learning difficulties, short attention span, and distractibility
  b. abdominal pain, vomiting, constipation, anorexia, headache, and fever

3. To refer the child immediately for examination and lead screening.

4.
  a. 20-44 µg/dl
  b. 45-69 µg/dl
  c. ≥ 70 µg/dl

5.
  a. removal of source of lead
  b. improving nutrition
  c. use of chelating therapy

6.
  a. Wash child's hands and face before eating.
  b. Run water for at least 2 minutes from *cold water* tap for drinking, cooking, and making formula.
  c. Do not store food in open cans, particularly if cans are imported.
  d. Make sure child eats regular meals, since more lead is absorbed on an empty stomach.

3. Make sure child's diet contains plenty of iron, calcium, protein, and zinc.

Section IV D

1.
  a. type of parenting received; negative relationship with own parents; low self-esteem; inadequate knowledge of normal development; concept of role reversal; lack of knowledge of parenting skills; social isolation
  b. temperament; position in the family; additional physical and/or emotional needs; activity level; illegitimacy; reminds parents of someone they dislike; prematurity; product of difficult delivery

c. chronic stress from divorce; financial deficits, unemployment; lack of support system; absence of a parent; alcoholism; drug addiction

2.

a. a thorough physical examination
b. detailed history

3.

a. conflicting stories about the accident or injury
b. an injury inconsistent with the history
c. history inconsistent with the child's developmental level
d. inappropriate response of caregiver
e. a complaint other than the obvious injury; excessive delay in seeking treatment
f. refusal of the parents to sign for additional tests

4.

a. Potential for trauma related to characteristics of child, caregiver(s), environment
b. Fear/anxiety related to negative interpersonal interaction, repeated maltreatment, powerless
c. Altered parenting related to child caregiver, or situational characteristics that precipitate abusive behavior

5. The record of the hospital admission or home visit may be important evidence of abuse.

6.

a. Victim is removed from environment.
b. Child is free of injury or neglect.
c. Child exhibits minimal or no evidence of distress.
d. Families exhibit evidence of positive interaction with children.
e. Parents demonstrate appropriate parenting activities.
f. Parents demonstrate an understanding of normal expectations for their child.

Chapter 15

Question   Answer

Section III

1. peer groups
2. first deciduous tooth; permanent teeth
3. F
4.

a. a decrease in head circumference in relation to standing height
b. a decrease in waist circumference in relation to height
c. an increase in leg length related to height.

5. 12;14
6. d
7. d
8. inferiority or inadequacy
9. T
10. c
11. T
12. Conservation
13. The ability to group objects according to the attributes they share
14. T
15. d
16. b
17. peers
18. F
19.

a. to appreciate the numerous and varied points of view that are represented in the peer group
b. to become increasingly sensitive to the social norms and pressure of the peer group
c. to form intimate friendships between same-sex peers

20. formalized groups; clubs
21. team games; sports
22.

a. modification of personal goals to group goals
b. the division of labor as an effective strategy for the attainment of a goal
c. the nature of competition and the importance of winning

23. a conscious awareness of a variety of self-perceptions, such as one's physical characteristics, abilities, values, and ideals and expectancy and one's idea of self in relation to others
24. family
25. teachers
26.

a. Meet the teacher at the beginning of school and plan to visit the school to see what is taught and expected.
b. Send the child to school every day - teachers are concerned when parents make other plans for their children; regular attendance conveys the impression that school is important.
c. Demonstrate an interest in what the child is learning.
d. Demonstrate an interest in content and growth more than in grades.

27. stomach pains or headaches, sleep problems, bed-wetting, changes in eating habits, aggressive or stubborn behavior, or reluctance to participate in activities
28.

a. easy availability of high-calorie foods
b. tendency toward more sedentary activities

29.
    a. a
    b. b
    c. b
    d. c
30. T
31.
    a. physiologic aspects of human sexuality
    b. cultural and societal values
    c. her own attitudes, feelings, and biases about sexuality
32. T

Section IV A

1.
    a. falls at the 50th percentile
    b. falls at the 50th percentile
2. At Jimmy's stage of development, he needs and wants real achievement. When he has access to tasks that need to be done, and is suitably rewarded, he will be able to achieve a sense of industry and accomplishment.
3. Lying, cheating, and stealing are frequent occurrences in the young school-age child. Children of this age do not understand why dishonesty is wrong. This behavior usually disappears as they mature.
4.
    a. Provide the child with support as unobtrusively as possible without feeling rejected, hurt, or angry.
    b. Respect the child's need for privacy and independence while maintaining limit-setting and discipline.
    c. Prepare the child for the body changes of pubescence.
    d. Make certain that the child's sex education is adequate and accurate.
    e. Allow for some regressive behavior.
    f. Reinforce earlier safety teaching.

Section IV B

1. The child needs to fit into a peer group and gain a sense of industry through individual, cooperative performance. It is necessary to move away from the familiar relationships of the family group to increase the scope of interpersonal interactions and explore the environment.
2. This is the first time that children are able to join in group activities with unrestrained enthusiasm and steady participation. Formerly, interactions were limited to short periods under considerable adult supervision.
3. It provides children with comfortable places in society.

Chapter 16

Question   Answer

Section III

1. secondary sex characteristics; body growth
2.
    a. the maturational, hormonal, and growth processes that occur when the reproductive organs begin to function and secondary sex characteristics develop
    b. means "to grow into maturity" and is generally regarded as the psychologic, social, and maturational process initiated by the pubertal changes
3. hormonal activity
4.
    a. increased physical growth
    b. appearance and development of secondary sex characteristics
5.
    a. the external and internal organs that carry on the reproductive functions
    b. changes that occur throughout the body as a result of the hormonal change
6. Estrogen; androgens
7. growth spurt
8. 10; 15; 12
9. nocturnal emissions
10. height; arms and legs; shoulder; hip development
11. T
12. Sebaceous; acne
13. T
14. b
15. group; personal
16. acceptance
17. When the individual is unable to formulate a satisfactory identity from the multiplicity of aspirations, roles, and identifications.
18. peers; adults
19. mature; childlike
20. formal operations
21.
    a. can think beyond the present
    b. is capable of formal logic
    c. is capable of mentally manipulating more than two categories of variables at the same time
    d. is able to detect logical inconsistencies and can evaluate a system of values in a more analytic manner
    e is to differentiate the thoughts of others from his own

22. peer group
23. 50%
24. same-gender
25. F
26.

    a. verbalize conceptually
    b. establish independence
    c. become comfortable with their bodies
    d. build new and meaningful relationships
    e. seek economic and social stability
    f. develop a workable value system

27. T
28.

    a. calcium
    b. iron
    c. zinc

29.

    a. growth and development
    b. education process
    c. better health

30. visual refractive difficulties
31.

    a. body image
    b. sexuality conflicts
    c. scholastic pressures
    d. competitive pressures
    e. relationship with parents
    f. relationship with siblings
    g. relationship with peers
    h. finances
    i. decisions about present and future roles
    j. career planning
    k. ideologic conflicts

32.

    a. biologic
    b. social
    c. health
    d. personal adjustment and attitudes
    e. interpersonal association
    f. establishment of values

33. physical injury
34. motor vehicle-related injury
35.

    a. inexperience
    b. lack of defensive driving skills
    c. alcohol and drug use

Section IV A

1.

    a. between the 50th and 75th percentile
    b. at the 95th percentile

2. Nonlean body mass, primarily fat, increases in adolescence. Fatty tissue deposition is more pronounced in girls, particularly in the regions over the thighs, hips, buttocks, and breast tissue. While the 95th percentile is the top of the normal range, nutritional counseling to prevent additional weight gain and/or eating disorders should be instituted.

Section IV B

1. A sense of group identity is essential to the later development of personal identity. Younger adolescents must resolve questions concerning relationships with a peer group before they are able to resolve questions about who they are in relation to the family and society.

2.

    a. wearing clothes, makeup, and hairstyles according to group criteria
    b. enjoying music and dancing that is exclusive to the age group
    c. using the same language
    d. conforming to the peer group rather than to the adult world

3. They serve as a strong support to the adolescent, individually and collectively, providing a sense of belonging and a feeling of strength and power. They form a transitional world between dependence and autonomy.

4.

    a. Adolescents are subject to turbulent, unpredictable behavior.
    b. Adolescents are struggling for independence.
    c. Adolescents are extremely sensitive to feelings and behavior that affect them.
    d. Adolescents may receive a different message than what was sent.
    e. Adolescents consider friends extremely important.
    f. Adolescents have a strong need "to belong."

Section IV C

1.

    a. necessary to support accelerated skeletal growth
    b. necessary for meeting the needs of increased muscle and soft-tissue growth and the demands of the expanding red cell mass
    c. essential for growth and sexual maturation

2. Rapid physical growth, increased activity, and a propensity for staying up late tend to contribute to this.

3.
   a. exercise for growing muscles
   b. interactions with peers
   c. socially acceptable means to enjoy stimulation and conflict
4. This is a period when orthodontic appliances are usually worn, so it is important to provide instructions regarding use and care of the appliances and emphasize attention to toothbrushing.
5.
   a. motor vehicle accidents
   b. drowning
   c. burns
   d. poisoning
   e. falls
   f. bodily damage
6. The need for independence, coupled with the propensity for risk taking and feelings of indestructibility, makes the adolescent vulnerable. The need for peer approval often causes the adolescent to attempt hazardous feats.
7.
   a. simple, correct explanations of sexual functions
   b. accurate information about pregnancy, including contraception
   c. the transmission, symptoms, and treatment of sexually transmitted diseases
   d. information about sexuality in the opposite sex
   e. reassurance regarding thoughts, fantasies, and masturbation
8.
   a. involve adolescent in diet planning; discuss four basic food groups and their importance in daily diet; associate proper diet with improved physical appearance
   b. educate to the need for sleep in proportion to physical activity; stress importance of a regular sleep pattern
   c. encourage participation in sports; educate to the release of tension through physical activity
   d. explain physical changes occurring in adolescence that require increased bathing and shampooing; assess knowledge of menstrual hygiene
   e. stress necessity of using car restraint systems; reinforce the dangers of drugs; discourage smoking; advise regarding excessive exposure to sunlight; encourage use of protective equipment; encourage practice of safety principles and prevention

Chapter 17

Question   Answer

Section III

1. Epstein-Barr virus
2.
   a. headache
   b. malaise
   c. fatigue
   d. chilliness
   e. low-grade fever
   f. loss of appetite
   g. puffy eyes
3. Monospot
4. imitation of adult behavior, peer pressure, and emulation of traits popularly attributed to smokers
5.
   a. preparation
   b. initiation
   c. experimentation
   d. regular smoking
6. F
7.
   a. peer-led programming
   b. use of media, such as videotapes and films
8. preparation and evaluation for activities; prevention of injury; treatment of injuries; rehabilitation after injury
9.
   a. "Little League elbow"
   b. "Tennis elbow"
   c. Osgood-Schlatter disease
10. repeated muscle contraction in repetitive weight-bearing sports
11.
   a. rest or alteration of activities
   b. physical therapies
   c. medication
12. T
13. inadequate nutrition
14.
   a. short stature
   b. sexual infantilism
   c. amenorrhea
15.
   a. tall with long legs
   b. small testes
   c. aberrant behavior
   d. defective development of secondary sex characteristics
   e. azoospermia
16. F

17. prostaglandins
18.
    a. infections
    b. hematuria
    c. penile problems, such as nonretractable foreskin in uncircumcised males; carcinoma; and trauma
    d. scrotal conditions, such as varicocele
    e. testicular torsion
19. to obtain medical care for her if she has not already done so.
20. suited to the individual
21.
    a. abstinence
    b. withdrawal
    c. rhythm
    d. barrier methods
    e. chemicals
    f. oral contraceptives
    g. implanted contraceptives
22. gonococcal; chlamydial
23.
    a. Herpes progenitalis
    b. Acquired immunodeficiency syndrome
24.
    a. 4, 11
    b. 1, 8
    c. 2, 9
    d. 5, 11
    e. 6, 10
    f. 3, 7
25. effects on the reproductive system, such as acute abcess formation in the fallopian tubes, chronic pelvic pain, dyspareunia, formation of adhesions, and increased risk for ectopic pregnancy
26. T
27.
    a. all right
    b. not being blamed for the situation
28.
    a. the acute phrase of disorganization of life style
    b. the long-term reorganization process
29. obesity
30. overweight
31. A caloric intake that consistently exceeds caloric requirements and expenditure
32.
    a. adipose cell theory
    b. set point theory
33. F
34.
    a. Modify diet to provide loss of fat content without interfering with growth, normal activity, and psychologic well-being
    b. Implement a regular exercise program

    c. Modify eating behavior
    d. Provide psychologic support
35. a
36. anorexia nervosa
37. menarche
38.
    a. upper or middle class
    b. academic high achievers
    c. conforming and conscientious
    d. high energy levels
    e. often described as "good children"
39.
    a. a relentless pursuit of thinness
    b. a fear of fatness
40.
    a. severe and profound weight loss
    b. signs of altered metabolic activity
    c. secondary or primary amenorrhea
    d. bradycardia
    e. lowered body temperature
    f. decreased blood pressure
    g. cold intolerance
    h. dry skin and brittle nails
    i. appearance of lanugo hair
41. Bulimia
42. self-induced vomiting, diuretics, laxatives
43.
    a. those who consume vast quantities of food followed by purging but who, if unable to purge, still eat large amounts
    b. those who restrict their caloric intake, especially when unable to purge
44. T
45.
    a. monitoring of fluid and electrolyte alterations
    b. observation for signs of cardiac complications
46. developmentally inappropriate degrees of inattention, impulsiveness, and hyperactivity
47.
    a. family education and counseling
    b. medication
    c. environmental manipulation
    d. remedial education
48. repeated involuntary urination (usually nocturnal) in children beyond the age when voluntary bladder control should normally have been acquired.
49.
    a. drugs
    b. bladder training
    c. restriction or elimination of fluids after evening meal
    d. interruption of sleep to void
    e. electrical devices
50. repeated voluntary or involuntary passage of feces of normal or near-normal consistency into

places not appropriate for that purpose according to the individual's own sociocultural setting.
51. idiopathic fecal incontinence (IFI)
52. inconsistent toilet training; psychosocial stress
53.
    a. initial response
    b. defense mechanisms are mobilized
    c. coping
54. to return the child to school
55. psychogenic
56. F
57.
    a. predominantly sad facial expression with absence or diminished range of affective response
    b. solitary play, work, or tendency to be alone; disinterest in play
    c. lowered grades in school; lack of interest in doing homework or achieving in school
    d. diminished motor activity; tiredness
    e. change in appetite resulting in weight loss or gain
    f. alterations in sleeping pattern
    g. tearfulness or crying
58. severe deviations
59. alcohol and cocaine
60. cocaine
61. assessment; function
62. T
63.
    a. act performed without any real attempt to cause either serious injury or death but rather to send a signal that something is wrong
    b. a deliberate act that is intended to cause injury or death
64. drug overdose
65. T
66.
    a. early recognition
    b. management
    c. prevention

Section IV A

1. On the basis of clinical manifestations, an absolute increase in atypical lymphocytes, a positive heterophil agglutination test, and a positive Monospot test.
2.
    a. disappear within 7 to 10 days
    b. subsides within 2 to 4 weeks
    c. usually 2 to 3 months
3. A short course of oral penicillin, gargles, hot drinks, analgesic troches, and mild analgesics
4.
    a. to relieve the symptoms

    b. to establish appropriate activities

Section IV B

1.
    a. acute overload
    b. chronic overload (overuse syndrome)
2. To alleviate the repetitive stress that initiated the symptoms
3. reduced activity and use of alternative exercise to keep the athlete mobile and maintain conditioning
4. Whether running provides both pleasure and physical benefits for him at the present time and into adulthood
5.
    a. collaborate with coaches to ensure safety measures
    b. assess for environmental safety risks
    c. counsel child and parents regarding the choice of appropriate sports activities
    d. recommend alternative activities when appropriate

Section IV C

1.
    a. infections, especially sexually transmitted diseases
    b. problems related to menstruation: delay, discomfort, or irregularities
2.
    a. the girls and her parents can be assured that her body is normal, contributing to a positive body image
    b. it provides an opportunity for health teaching in the areas of hygiene, body functions, and sexuality
    c. it provides an opportunity for the girl to ask questions about her changing body and the implications of those changes
    d. if any reproductive system problems arise during adolescence, experience makes the exam less stressful
3.
    a. the delay of menarche beyond the age of 17
    b. absence of menstruation for 12 months or more between periods in the first 2 years following menarche or when more than three periods have been missed following the establishment of menses
4.
    a. endometriosis
    b. pelvic inflammatory disease

Section IV D

1. A period of a year or two of mood disturbances and behavior changes. The weight loss may be triggered by an adolescent crisis such as the onset of menstruation or a traumatic interpersonal incident.
2.
    a. The current emphasis on slimness as a standard for beauty and femininity
    b. Increased family stress
3.
    a. B
    b. A, B
    c. A
    d. B
    e. A
    f. A
    g. B
    h. A, B
    i. B
    j. B
    k. A, B
    l. A
4.
    a. consistency
    b. teamwork
    c. continuity
    d. communication
    e. support of client, family, and staff

Section IV E

1. Because it is obvious to others, is difficult to treat, and has long-term effects on psychologic and physical health status
2.
    a. genetic
    b. diseases
    c. metabolic and endocrine disturbances
    d. caloric disequilibrium
    e. cellular structure
    f. psychologic, social, and cultural
3.
    a. eat more at a given sitting than nonobese persons
    b. eat more rapidly than nonobese persons
    c. overeat when they are not hungry
    d. tend to "gorge" at one meal, rather than eating intermittently over time
    e. tend to be night eaters
    f. often skip meals, particularly breakfast
4.
    a. altered nutrition: more than body requirements related to obesity and overweight
    b. activity intolerance related to sedentary lifestyle, physical bulk

c. ineffective individual coping related to little or no exercise, poor nutrition, personal vulnerability
d. self-esteem disturbance related to perception of physical appearance, internalization of negative feedback
e. altered family processes related to management of child who is obese

Section IV F

1. An impulsive act designed to punish or manipulate a loved person perceived as withdrawing that love
2. Girls make more unsuccessful suicide attempts than boys and are likely to ingest pills as the method.
3. A disturbed family situation, such as economic stresses, family disintegration, medical problems, psychiatric illness, abandonment, or alcoholism

Chapter 18

Question   **Answer**

Section III

1.
    a. 3
    b. 1
    c. 4
    d. 2
2. T
3.
    a. developmental focus = focus on the child's developmental age rather than chronologic age or diagnosis
    b. family-centered care = a philosophy of care that recognizes the family as the constant in a child's life and that service systems and personnel must support, respect, encourage, and enhance the strength and competence of the family
    c. Normalization = establishing a normal pattern of living
4. Mainstreaming
5.
    a. losing a perfect child
    b. adjusting to and accepting the child and his condition
6.
    a. shock and denial
    b. adjustment
    c. reintegration and acknowledgment
    d. freezing-out phase

7.
  a. guilt
  b. anger

8.
  a. the parents fear letting the child achieve any new skill, avoid all discipline, and cater to every desire to prevent frustration
  b. the parents detach themselves emotionally from the child but usually provide adequate physical care or constantly nag and scold the child
  c. the parents act as if the disorder does not exist or attempt to have the child overcompensate for it
  d. the parents place necessary and realistic restrictions on the child, encourage self-care activities, and promote reasonable physical and social abilities

9. Chronic sorrow is an emotional response that is manifested throughout the life span of the parent/child interaction. Acceptance is interspersed with periods of intensified sorrow for the loss, especially at ceratin landmarks of the child's development.

10. a couple's marital functioning before the birth or diagnosis of a child with special needs

11. T

12. feelings, perceptions, reactions

13.
  a. available support systems
  b. perception of the event
  c. coping mechanisms

14.
  a. denial
  b. anger
  c. bargaining
  d. depression
  e. acceptance

15.
  a. shock and disbelief
  b. expression of grief
  c. disorganization and despair
  d. reorganization

16.
  a. the child's developmental level
  b. available coping mechanisms
  c. the reactions of significant others to him
  d. the condition itself

17. T

18.
  a. develops competence and optimism
  b. feels different and withdraws
  c. is irritable, moody, and acts out
  d. complies with treatment
  e. seeks support

19. T

20. 9 or 10 years old

21. separation from parents

22.
  a. congenital anomaly
  b. cognitive impairment
  c. physical disability
  d. chronic illness
  e. multiple disabilities
  f. terminal illness

23.
  a. denial
  b. guilt
  c. anger

24.
  a. preparation
  b. participation
  c. sharing
  d. control
  e. expectation

25.
  a. information regarding the disorder
  b. developmental needs of the child
  c. realistic goal setting

26.
  a. Do you have a good social support system?
  b. Do you have a good professional support system?
  c. Do you maintain good health practices?
  d. Do you use distancing techniques?
  e. Can you focus on the positive aspects of the caregiving role?
  f. Can you reflect on positive feedback from appreciative families?

Section IV A

1.
  a. care is now focused on the child's developmental age rather than chronologic age
  b. care is now focused on family-centered care
  c. increased use of the principle of normalization
  d. tend toward mainstreaming, or integrating children with special needs into a regular classroom

2.
  a. Using the developmental approach emphasizes the child's abilities and strengths rather than his disability. Under the developmental model, attention is directed to the child's functional development, changes, and adaptation to the environment.
  b. Families are supported in their natural caregiving and decision-making roles by building on their unique strengths as individuals and families.
  c. By applying the principles of normalization,

the environment for the child is "normalized" and "humanized."

  d. The school has now become an essential component of the child's overall physical, intellectual, and social development

Section IV B

1.
  a. to provide emotional support to the family
  b. to anticipate and prevent potential problems
  c. to foster growth despite the disorder

2.
  a. this is a period of intense emotion and is characterized by shock, disbelief, and sometimes denial, especially if the disorder is not obvious.
  b. this follows shock and is usually characterized by an open admission that the condition exists. This stage is manifested by several responses such as guilt and anger.
  c. this stage is characterized by realistic expectations for the child and reintegration of family life, with the child's condition in proper perspective. The family also broadens its activities to include relationships outside the home, with the child being an acceptable and participating member of the group.
  d. not all families reach the stage of acceptance and reintegration. If strategies of coping can't be employed to minimize the stress and disorganization of maintaining the child within the home, the child may be placed outside the home.

3.
  a. shopping for physicians
  b. attributing the symptoms of the actual illness to a minor condition
  c. refusal to believe the diagnostic tests
  d. delay in agreeing to treatment
  e. acting very happy and optimistic despite the revealed diagnosis
  f. refusing to tell or talk to anyone about the condition
  g. insisting that no one is telling the truth regardless of others' attempts to do so
  h. denying the reason for admission
  i. asking no questions about the diagnosis, treatment, or prognosis

4.
  a. It allows individuals to distance themselves from the onslaught of a tremendous emotional impact and to collect and mobilize their energies toward goal-directed, problem-solving behaviors.
  b. It allows the individual to maintain hope in the face of overwhelming odds.

5.
  a. in addition to grieving for the loss of a perfect child, they are less likely to receive positive feedback from transactions with their child. Parenting such children may be a series of unrewarding experiences, which continually support the parents' feelings of inadequacy and failure. Excessive demands on parents' time place additional strain on the couple. This may lead to feelings of resentment, anger, and bitterness toward the other for having their life-style disrupted by the child's condition.
  b. Most siblings experience mixed feelings. They may feel left out, guilt, sadness, shame, resentment, jealousy, anger, pride, and love.

Section IV C

1.
  a. status of the marital relationship
  b. alternate support systems
  c. ability to communicate

2. This aids in evaluating the individual's ability to cope with various aspects of the crisis and identifies possible areas for intervention.

3.
  a. child identifies own assets and strengths realistically
  b. child verbalizes positive suggestions for adjusting to the disability
  c. child becomes involved with special group activities

4.
  a. provide support at the time of diagnosis
  b. educate the family about child's condition
  c. accept the family's emotional reactions
  d. help the family cope
  e. promote normal development

5.
  a. family's available support system
  b. family's perception of the illness or disability
  c. family's knowledge of the condition
  d. influence of religion on their thinking
  e. current stresses on family
  f. family's reactions to the child

6.
  a. provide accurate information in language that the parents can understand; provide guidance in how the condition may interfere with activities of daily living; stress the importance of communicating the child's condition in the event of a medical emergency; provide information about child's condition and therapeutic plan; and provide

information regarding sexuality in relation to disability.
   b. help the child realize his potential in preparation for the next phase of development; evaluate the child's developmental progress at regular intervals; teach parents successful methods of controlling behaviors before they become problems
   c. encourage the parents to determine realistic expectations for the child; encourage genetic counseling; encourage independence

Section IV D

1.
   a. They see death as a departure.
   b. They may recognize the fact of physical death but do not separate it from living abilities.
   c. They view death as temporary and gradual.
2. as punishment for his thoughts or actions
3. 9; 10
4. because, developmentally, the adolescent's task is to establish an identity by finding out who he is, what his purpose is, and where he belongs. Any suggestion of being different or nonbeing is a tremendous threat to the answers to such questions. The adolescent's concern is for the present much more than the past or the future.
5.
   a. help parents deal with their feelings, allowing them more emotional reserve to meet the needs of their children
   b. avoid alliances with either parent or child
   c. structure the hospital admission to allow for maximum self-control and independence
   d. answer the adolescent's questions honestly, treating them as mature individuals
   e. help parents understand their child's reactions to death/dying

Section IV E

1.
   a. In this first stage, the family responds with shock and disbelief.
   b. When denial fails and the reality of the situation penetrates the consciousness, the family's reaction is "Why did this happen to my child?"
   c. attempt to postpone the inevitable. Bargaining may be with God, with oneself, or with the most significant other person
   d. Generally, there are two types of depression: the type experienced for past losses, and the type experienced for anticipated or impending losses.

   e. This is the final stage of dying. The family is no longer angry or depressed, and if bargaining occurs, it is usually for a peaceful, painless death rather than for prolongation of life.
2. Parents may experience more guilt, a prolonged period of numbness and shock, intense loneliness and emptiness, anxious fear that someone else will die and intense anger. Family is denied the opportunity to complete all "unfinished business" and to prepare for and begin the grief process. Guilt and remorse for not having done something additional or different with the child can be overwhelming.

Section IV F

1.
   a. promote self-help (self-care)
   b. enhance child's sense of competence and mastery
2.
   a. provide opportunity for family to adjust to discovery of diagnosis
   b. anticipate the usual grief reaction to loss of "perfect" child
   c. explore family's feeling regarding the child and their ability to cope with the disorder
   d. encourage family to express their concerns
   e. repeat information as often as necessary
   f. serve as role model regarding attitudes and behavior toward the child
3. altered growth and development related to chronic illness, parental reactions, and repeated hospitalization.

Section IV G

1.
   a. support child during terminal phase
   b. provide physical comfort and nurturing at time of dying
   c. provide emotional support at time of dying
2.
   a. child expresses feelings freely
   b. child demonstrates an understanding of symptoms

Chapter 19

Question   Answer

Section III

1. Cognitive impairments
2. Significantly subaverage general intellectual functioning existing concurrently with deficits in adaptive behavior and manifested during the developmental period.
3. It implies that intelligence alone is not the criterion for mental retardation.
4. after a period of suspicion by professionals and/or the family that the child's developmental progress is delayed.
5. standard intelligence tests
6.
  a. genetic
  b. biochemical
  c. viral
  d. developmental
7.
  a. infection and intoxication
  b. trauma or physical agents
  c. metabolism or nutritional deficiencies
  d. gross postnatal brain disease
  e. unknown prenatal influences
  f. conditions such as prematurity, low birth weight, and postmaturity that originate in the perinatal period
  g. psychiatric disorders
  h. environmental influences
  i. chromosomal abnormalities
8. This act requires local departments of education to provide education programs for handicapped children 3 years of age or older.
9.
  a. a task analysis of the individual steps needed to master a skill must be done before teaching
  b. sequencing of skills taught must be guided by normal sequence of development
10. recreational and educational value.
11. Safety
12. Down syndrome
13. 21
14. through a chromosomal analysis
15. F
16. Hypotonicity of chest and abdominal muscles
17.
  a. indicates disability that may range in severity from mild to profound and includes the subsets of deaf and hard-of-hearing
  b. refers to a person whose hearing disability precludes successful processing of linguistic information through audition, with or without a hearing aid
  c. a person who, generally with the use of a hearing aid, has residual hearing sufficient to enable successful processing of linguistic information through audition
18.
  a. family history
  b. anatomic malformation of head or neck
  c. low birth weight
  d. severe perinatal asphyxia
  e. perinatal infection (cytomegalovirus, rubella, herpes, syphilis, toxoplasmosis, bacterial meningitis)
  f. chronic ear infection
  g. cerebral palsy
  h. Down syndrome
  i. ototoxic drugs
19.
  a. 1, 4, 6, 10
  b. 2, 7, 9, 11
  c. 1, 3
  d. 5, 8
20.
  a. an inability to express ideas in any form, either written or verbal
  b. the inability to interpret sound correctly
  c. difficulty in processing details of or discriminating among sounds
21. according to the degree of severity of loss
22. decibel
23. acoustic feedback
24. when there is visual acuity of 20/200 or less and/or a visual field of 20 degrees or less in the better eye
25. Refractive errors
26. This refers to variations within the eye that prevent perfect focusing of light rays on the retina.
27. T
28.
  a. 2, 8
  b. 1, 7, 10
  c. 5, 9
  d. 3, 6
29. This is a reduced visual acuity in one eye, despite appropriate optical correction that occurs in the absence of any pathologic defect in the affected eye. It is also referred to as "lazy eye."
30. The optimum time for correction is during early childhood. Treatment consists of patching the "good eye" so that the child will be forced to use the weaker eye. If refractive errors are present, corrective lenses are worn.
31. Strabismus
32. When there is malalignment, the eyes see two

separate images (diplopia). Because the brain suppresses the images from the weaker or deviating eye, amblyopia can result in children under 9 years of age.

33. esotropic
34.
   a. an opacity of the crystalline lens
   b. a condition in which intraocular pressure is increased, causing pressure on the optic nerve and eventually atrophy and blindness
35. because motor development is very dependent on sight
36. loss of sight and hearing
37. They interfere with the normal sequence of physical, intellectual, and psychosocial growth.
38. retinoblastoma
39. 90%

Section IV A

1. optimum medical care
2. promoting the child's optimum development as an individual within a family and community
3. his learning abilities and deficits
4.
   a. developmental age
   b. functional level of self-help activities
   c. any special needs the child may have
   d. unusual or favorite routines
   e. any behaviors that may require intervention
5.
   a. ensure that the child has appropriate toys to entertain him
   b. place the child in a room with other children of approximately the same developmental age
   c. treat the child with dignity and respect
   d. explain procedures to the child using methods of communication appropriate for his cognitive level
   e. focus on growth-promoting experiences for the child

Section IV B

1.
   a. varies from severely retarded to low-normal intelligence, but is generally within the mild to moderate range; initial development may appear near normal although slowed development, especially in speech, is characteristic
   b. growth in both height and weight reduced; obesity common. Sexual development delayed, incomplete, or both. Males infertile; females can be fertile. Premature aging common; lowered life expectancy.
   c. congenital heart disease is common; other

structural defects include renal agenesis, duodenal atresia, Hirschsprung disease, tracheoesophageal fistula; skeletal defects.
   d. visual problems include strabismus, myopia, nystagmus, cataracts, or conjunctivitis; conductive hearing loss occurs in a large percentage
   e. respiratory infections are very prevalent
2.
   a. ensuring that the parents are informed as soon as possible following the birth of the child
   b. encouraging parents to be together at this time to emotionally support each other
   c. providing parents with written material concerning the syndrome
   d. discussing with parents the benefits of home care versus institutional care
   e. providing parents with available sources of assistance

Section IV C

1. He is often unable to proceed past parallel play within a group because of his inability to follow directions during cooperative play. Also, his deficit may not allow him to interpret enough of the conversation to join in. As a result, he learns to stay on the periphery or to avoid social interactions altogether.
2.
   a. treat existing ear infections and prevent recurrences; encourage periodic auditory testing for children at risk; stress the need for routine immunizations; administer ototoxic agents cautiously; counsel pregnant women regarding the necessity of early prenatal care; prevent exposure to excessive noise.
   b. screen all children for auditory function; observe for behaviors that indicate a hearing loss.
3.
   a. lack of startle reflex to a loud sound; failure to be awakened by loud environmental noises; failure to localize a source of sound by 6 months of age; absence of babble or inflections in voice by age 7 months; general indifference to sound; lack of response to the spoken word; response to loud noises as opposed to the voice.
   b. use of gestures rather than verbalization; failure to develop intelligible speech by age 24 months; vocal play, head banging, foot stamping; yelling or screeching to express pleasure; asking to have statements repeated; shyness, timidity, withdrawal.
4. mild = clear but loud; monotone voice; difficulty in articulation

severe = failure to babble or develop intelligible speech; unintelligible speech; yelling or screeching
5. because speech is learned through a multisensory approach and the usual mechanisms are not available to the deaf child
6.
   a. promote independence and development
   b. provide opportunities for play and socialization
   c. encourage education within a regular classroom

Section IV D

1.
   a. support the child and family
   b. promote parent-child attachment
   c. promote the child's optimum development
   d. care for the child during hospitalization
   e. assist in measures to prevent vision impairment
2.
   a. avoid excessive eyestrain; when doing close work, periodically look into the distance to relax the muscles of accommodation
   b. use proper lighting; light should not be glaring or cast shadows on reading material
   c. get sufficient amounts of rest and nutrition
   d. have eyes checked at least yearly by a licensed optometrist or ophthalmologist
   e. teach safety regarding common eye injuries
3.
   a. help parents identify clues other than eye contact from the infant that signify communication
   b. encourage parents to discuss their feelings regarding lack of visual contact or smiling from the child
   c. stress that the lack of such responses is not an indication of child's rejection or dislike of parents
   d. demonstrate by own example acceptance of the child
   e. emphasize positive abilities or attributes
   f. encourage parents in their attempt to promote child's development

Section IV E

1.
   a. identify the signs of retinoblastoma
   b. prepare the family for diagnostic/therapeutic procedures and home care
   c. provide emotional support to the child and his family
2.
   a. observe for signs of retinoblastoma
   b. explain to parents about the procedures performed and the expected reactions of their child

c. encourage parents to seek genetic counseling for themselves and for the child after he reaches puberty

Chapter 20

Question	Answer

Section III

1.
   a. developmental age
   b. previous experience with illness, separation, or hospitalization
   c. available support system
   d. innate and acquired coping skills
   e. seriousness of diagnosis
2. Separation
3. protest; despair; detachment (or denial)
4. peers
5. physical restriction; altered routine or rituals; dependency
6.
   a. 1
   b. 2
   c. 2
   d. 1
   e. 3
   f. 4
   g. 1
   h. 4
   i. 3
   j. 2
7. 6 months
8.
   a. T
   b. F
   c. T
   d. F
   e. T
   f. T
   g. F
9.
   a. "difficult" temperament
   b. poor child-parent relationship
   c. age (especially between 6 months and 5 years)
   d. male gender
   e. below-average intelligence
   f. multiple and continuing stresses
10. F
11. Pain is whatever the experiencing person says it is, existing whenever the person says it does.

12.
  a. infants and children do not feel pain or feel pain less than adults do.
  b. children cannot tell where they hurt
  c. children always tell the truth about their pain
  d. children tolerate pain better than adults and become accustomed to pain or painful procedures
  e. behavioral manifestations of pain reflect pain intensity
  f. narcotics are dangerous drugs for children. They cause addiction and respiratory depression.

13.
  a. question the child
  b. use pain rating scales
  c. evaluate behavior and physiologic changes
  d. secure parents' involvement
  e. take cause of pain into account
  f. take action and evaluate results

14.
  a. faces scale
  b. oucher
  c. numeric scale
  d. poker chip
  e. color tool
  f. word graphic rating scale
  g. visual analogue scale

15. Fear of the unknown (fantasy) exceeds fear of the known

16.
  a. c
  b. c
  c. c
  d. x

17. patient-controlled analgesia (PCA)
18. respiratory depression
19. work
20. parent-child relationships; educational opportunities; self-mastery; socialization

21.
  a. disbelief
  b. anger; guilt
  c. fear; anxiety; frustration
  d. depression

22. anger; jealousy; resentment
23. isolation

24.
  a. physical stressors
  b. environmental stressors
  c. psychologic stressors
  d. social stressors

Section IV A

1. protest
2.
  a. allow the child to cry
  b. provide support through physical presence in room even when child rejects strangers
  c. acknowledge to the child that it is all right to miss her parents and it is all right to cry
  d. encourage parents to stay with the child as much as possible

Section IV B

1.
  a. Encourage parents to room-in.
  b. Encourage parents to participate in the care of the child.
  c. Assign a consistent primary nurse to care for Amy.
  d. Accept Amy's separation behavior.
  e. Help parents to understand Amy's separation behavior.
  f. Ask parents to bring some of the child's favorite toys and articles to the hospital.

2.
  a. Use the minimum amount of restraint of physical activity.
  b. Set schedules and routines as close to that of the child as possible.
  c. Decrease dependency of the child by allowing the child to do things for herself and allowing the child to make decisions.

Section IV C

1.
  a. encourage parents to participate
  b. provide support
  c. supply information
  d. prepare for discharge and home care

2.
  a. respect parental rights
  b. convey an attitude of respectful caring for both child and family
  c. support and emphasize the family's strengths and abilities
  d. provide feedback and praise
  e. refer to other professionals for additional support

3.
  a. recognize that family members know the child best and are "cued in" to the child's needs
  b. welcome unlimited family presence

c. encourage family to bring other significant family members to visit

d. encourage family to provide the child with significant, but manageable, items from home.

4. large puzzles, blocks, dress-up materials, puppets, scissors and paper, and crayons.

Section IV D

1.
   a. take a nursing admission history
   b. perform a physical assessment
   c. assess variables influencing placement of the child on the unit

2.
   a. be positive in your approach to the child
   b. be honest with the child
   c. convey to the child the behaviors expected
   d. be consistent in expectations and relationships with the child
   e. treat the child fairly and help the child to feel this
   f. encourage parents to maintain a truthful relationship with the child
   g. make certain the child has a call light or other signal device within reach

Chapter 21

Question   Answer

Section III

1. The legal and ethical requirement that the patient clearly, fully, and completely understands the medical treatment performed and all risks, consequences, or results that may or may not occur from medical treatment.

2.
   a. The person must be capable of giving consent, must be over the age of majority, and must be considered competent.
   b. The person must receive the information needed to make an intelligent decision.
   c. The person must act voluntarily when exercising freedom of choice without force, fraud, deceit, duress, or other forms of constraint or coercion.

3.
   a. one who is legally under age but is recognized as having the legal capacity of an adult under circumstances prescribed by law; for example, marriage
   b. one who has attained the specific age (usually 15 or 16) at which a minor may consent to medical or surgical treatment without parental consent; for example, contraceptive services, as long as they understand the consequences

4. preparation

5.
   a. child's developmental level
   b. child's cognitive ability
   c. child's temperament
   d. child's existing coping strategies
   e. child's previous experiences

6. F

7.
   a. expect success
   b. involve the child
   c. provide distraction
   d. allow expression of feelings

8.
   a. teach
   b. express feelings
   c. achieve a therapeutic goal

9.
   a. admission
   b. blood test
   c. afternoon of the day before surgery
   d. injection of preoperative medications
   e. before and during transport to OR
   f. return from the recovery room

10. 2

11. the extent to which the patient's behavior coincides with the prescribed regimen

12.
   a. clinical judgment
   b. self-reporting
   c. direct observation
   d. monitoring appointments
   e. monitoring therapeutic response
   f. pill counts
   g. chemical assay

13.
   a. organizational strategies
   b. educational strategies
   c. behavioral strategies

14. widely spaced teeth; pomade

15. avoided; osmotic

16.
   a. vomiting or diarrhea
   b. decrease in appetite
   c. abdominal cramping or distention
   d. absence of bowel sounds
   e. dehydration or weight loss

17. fever

18.
   a. c
   b. a
   c. b

19. antipyretics
20. increase
21.

   a. category-specific isolation precautions
   b. disease-specific isolation precautions
22. handwashing
23. time-out
24.

   a. age
   b. condition
   c. destination
25. restraints
26. glucose, ketones, protein, blood, bilirubin, urobilinogen, nitrates, potassium, creatinine, and urea.
27. the nurse must cleanse the genital area for the child instead of the child doing it himself. The nurse may hold the child over a sterile container, or she may apply a sterile plastic collecting bag. The start and stopping of urine stream (midstream) usually is impossible.
28. skin prep
29. body weight
30. check his hospital identification band
31.

   a. vastus lateralis muscle
   b. ventrogluteal muscle
32.

   a. amount of drug to be administered
   b. minimum dilution of drug
   c. type of solution in which drug can be diluted
   d. length of time over which drug can be safely administered
   e. rate of infusion that child and vessels can tolerate safely
   f. time that this or another drug is to be administered
   g. compatibility of all drugs that child is receiving intravenously
33.

   a. appropriately diluted medication is injected into the tubing at the site of the Y connection or through a stopcock in the direction of the child.
   b. appropriately diluted medication is injected into the IV tubing at site of the Y connection or stopcock in the direction away from the child.
34. venous access devices
35.

   a. Hickman/Broviac catheter
   b. Groshong catheter
   c. Implanted ports
36. as soon as possible after becoming soiled
37. they can accurately infuse fluids
38. retina, lungs

39.

   a. pulse oximetry
   b. transcutaneous monitoring (TCM)
40.

   a. effective in depositing medication directly into the airway
   b. avoids the systemic side effects of certain drugs
   c. reducing the amount of drug necessary to achieve the desired effect
41. T
42. chest physiotherapy
43. humidified
44. restlessness, dyspnea, pallor or cyanosis, changes in pulse or blood pressure, overt bleeding from trachea or around incision site, retractions, and noisy respirations
45. 0.5 cm.
46. only as often as necessary to keep the tube patent.
47. method using height as predictor of gastric tube insertion distance
48. button; gastroport
49. intravenous alimentation; hyperalimentation therapy.
50. rapid fluid shift and fluid overload
51.

   a. osmotic effect of the enema may produce diarrhea, which can lead to metabolic acidosis
   b. extreme hyperphosphatemia, hypernatremia, hypocalcemia, which may lead to neuromuscular irritability and coma, may occur
52. peristomal skin

Section IV A

1.

   a. The nurse who explains the procedure should be the one who supports the child throughout the procedure.
   b. Assemble all equipment before beginning procedure.
   c. Do not perform procedure in a "safe" room.
   d. Avoid lengthy conversation during procedure.
   e. Inform child when procedure is nearing completion.

Section IV B

1.

   a. ensure legal authorization
   b. provide hygienic preparation
   c. provide physical preparation
   d. prevent complications
   e. ensure safety

f. prepare to receive child upon return from surgery

2.

 a. institute preoperative teaching
 b. orient child to strange surroundings
 c. explain where parents will be while child is in operating room

3.

 a. child exhibits no evidence of dehydration
 b. child takes and retains fluids when allowed

Section IV C

1. Measure the rectal temperature 30 minutes after the antipyretic is given to assess whether the temperature is lowered.
2. Use minimum clothing, expose skin to air, reduce room temperature, increase air circulation, administer cool applications to the skin or give a cooling bath.
3. crib sides

Section IV D

1.

 a. increasing nutritional and fluid intake
 b. how to decrease elevated temperature
 c. safety concerns
 d. infection control
 e. play
2. Toys must be safe, appropriate to child's developmental level and condition.

Section IV E

1.

 a. provides a snug fit with minimum danger of becoming too tight
 b. prevents muscle injury and psychologic stress

Section IV F

1.

 a. Use a small amount of liquid or food—the child may refuse to take the entire amount and thus receive only a partial dose of the medication.
 b. Avoid essential food items—child may become conditioned against them and refuse these foods.

Section IV G

1.

 a. allow Mariano to see that there is always someone nearby
 b. allow him to have a favorite toy inside the tent
 c. if he is well enough, remove Mariano from the tent for feeding and bathing
 d. reassure him that he will not be left alone
2. this minimizes the chance of vomiting
3. you would auscultate the chest before treatment and then after treatment to hear whether the chest sounds clearer

Section IV H

1.

 a. change dressing around stoma three times a day
 b. maintain aseptic technique
 c. suction frequently
 d. keep an extra tracheostomy set at the bedside
 e. check patency of tube frequently by auscultation of the chest
 f. monitor the child for problems such as pallor, cyanosis, changes in pulse and/or blood pressure, and bleeding around the site
2. noisy breathing, bubbling, or coughing

Section IV I

1.

 a. because this entry causes less distress (since infants are obligatory nose breathers) and helps stimulate sucking.
 b. so that the fluid and electrolyte balance won't be upset by removing the fluids and electrolytes
 c. because of possible damage to the nostril
 d. to clear formula from the tube and prevent souring
 e. to minimize the possibility of regurgitation and aspiration

2.

 a. attaching a syringe to the feeding tube and attempting to aspirate stomach contents.
 b. with the syringe, injecting 0.5 ml of air into the tube while listening with a stethoscope to the stomach area for sounds of gurgling or growling. Withdrawn air.

3.

 a. return residual aspirated fluid to the stomach
 b. provide a pacifier during feeding

Chapter 22

Question   Answer

Section III

1. Respiratory failure
2.
   a. nature of the infectious agent
   b. age of the child
   c. resistance of natural defenses
   d. size and frequency of dose
   e. size of child
   f. presence of general conditions
   g. presence of disorders that affect the respiratory tract
3. viruses
4. The diameter of the respiratory tract is similar and therefore subject to narrowing from edema
5.
   a. T
   b. T
   c. F
   d. T
   e. F
   f. T
   g. F
   h. T
6. Saline nose drops
7. The moisture soothes inflamed membranes and assists in liquefying secretions.
8. using a hot shower for a few minutes
9. symptomatic
10. Depression of the cough reflex may increase the risk of aspiration.
11. Group A hemolytic streptococcus.
12. throat culture
13. an antibiotic for at least 10 days
14. to filter and protect the respiratory and the alimentary tracts from invasion by pathogenic organisms
15. palatine tonsils
16. adenoids
17. inflammation; swallowing; breathing
18. blockage of the eustachian tube, which interferes with normal drainage and frequently results in otitis media and difficulty in hearing
19.
   a. a child has massive hypertrophy that results in difficulty eating or extreme discomfort when breathing
   b. a child has recurrent otitis media, especially when associated with hearing loss and in those children where hypertrophied adenoids obstruct nasal breathing

20.
   a. blood loss may be excessive
   b. possibility of regrowth or hypertrophy of lymphoid tissue
21. monitoring vital signs, observing for hemorrhage, and assessing general response to surgery
22. for the first 24 hours
23. hemorrhage
24.
   a. an inflammation of the middle ear without reference to etiology or pathogenesis
   b. a rapid and short onset of signs and symptoms lasting approximately 3 weeks
   c. an inflammation of the middle ear in which a collection of fluid is present in the middle ear space
   d. middle ear effusion lasting from 3 weeks to 3 months
   e. middle ear effusion that persists beyond 3 months
25. *Streptococcus pneumoniae*; *Hemophilus influenzae*; *Staphylococcus aureus*
26. blocked eustachian tubes
27. hearing loss
28. intact membrane that appears bright red and bulging, with no visible landmarks or light reflex
29. amoxicillin; ampicillin
30. hearing impairment
31. Tympanostomy tubes
32. the primary anatomic area affected
33. laryngeal obstruction
34. airway; adequate respiratory exchange
35. to liquefy respiratory secretions and decrease edema of the respiratory tract
36. an obstructive inflammatory process
37. cherry-red edematous
38. it could precipitate a complete obstruction
39. Respiratory syncytial virus (RSV)
40. a narrowing of the respiratory passages on expiration, which prevents the air from leaving the lungs
41. viruses, bacteria, mycoplasmas; pneumonia associated with aspiration of foreign substances
42. the clinical history, the child's age, the child's general health history, the physical examination, radiography, and the laboratory examination
43. *Mycobacterium tuberculosis*
44. physical examination; history; reaction to tuberculin tests; radiographic examinations; isolation of tubercle bacilli by culture from sputum, gastric washings, and/or pleural fluid
45. chemotherapy

46.
   a. Isoniazid (INH)
   b. Rifampin (RMP)
   c. Pyrazinamide
47. avoid contact; Bacillus Calmette-Guerin
48. they are naturally curious and tend to put everything in their mouths
49. choking, gagging, wheezing, or cough
50. laryngoscopy; bronchoscopy
51. back blows; Heimlich maneuver
52. cannot speak; becomes cyanotic; collapses
53. secondary bacterial infection
54. prevention of aspiration
55.
   a. local
   b. systemic
56. carbon monoxide
57. 100% oxygen
58. Passive smoking
59. is a reversible obstructive process characterized by an increased responsiveness of the airway, especially the lower airways
60. allergic hypersensitivity to foreign substances
61.
   a. edema of mucous membranes
   b. accumulation of tenacious secretions from mucous glands
   c. spasm of the smooth muscle of the bronchi and bronchioles, which decreases the caliber of the bronchioles
62. Gas trapping; higher and higher lung volume
63.
   a. shortness of breath
   b. wheezing
   c. cough
64. prevent disability; minimize physical and psychologic morbidity
65. Allergen
66. control the acute attack; maximum
67. Rapid-acting bronchodilators
68.
   a. beta-adrenergics
   b. methylxanthines
69. methylxanthine
70. It has been found that moderate exercise or even strenuous exercise is advantageous for children with asthma.
71.
   a. breathing exercises
   b. physical training
   c. inhalation therapy
72. children who continue to display respiratory distress despite vigorous therapeutic measures
73. epinephrine
74.
   a. Asthma is a very common disease and to

have asthma is not disgraceful.
   b. Persons with asthma are able to live full and active lives.
   c. An asthmatic attack is easier to prevent than treat.
   d. Individuals do not become addicted to asthma medication, but they do prefer to breathe more freely whenever possible.
75. multisystem disorder primarily affecting the exocrine glands
76. autosomal-recessive trait
77. mechanical obstruction caused by the increased viscosity of mucous gland secretions
78. Pulmonary complications
79. Because essential pancreatic enzymes are unable to reach the duodenum, digestion and absorption of nutrients are markedly impaired.
80. meconium ileus
81. large, frothy, and extremely foul smelling
82.
   a. history of the disease in the family
   b. absence of pancreatic enzymes
   c. increase in electrolyte concentration of sweat
   d. chronic pulmonary involvement
83. sweat test
84. higher in calories, no restriction on fats, vitamins A, D, and E must be supplemented
85. improve pulmonary function and loosen and eliminate bronchial secretions
86.
   a. chest physiotherapy
   b. breathing exercises
   c. aerosol therapy
87. pulmonary involvement

Section IV A

1.
   a. ineffective breathing pattern caused by inflammatory process, pain
   b. ineffective airway clearance related to the inflammatory process
   c. fear/anxiety related to hospitalization, difficulty breathing
   d. pain related to inflammatory process
   e. potential for injury related to presence of infective organisms
   f. altered family process related to illness and/or hospitalization of child
   g. altered body temperature related to the inflammatory process
   h. altered nutrition: less than body requirements related to difficulty swallowing and loss of appetite

Section IV B

1. child would be irritable and pull on her ears or roll her head from side to side; she may have fever of as much as 104° F and signs of respiratory or pharyngeal infection; anorexia, crying, and purulent discharge may be present.
2. maintain regularity of administration of antibiotic and continue therapy for at least 10 days

Section IV C

1. monitor respirations; auscultate lungs; observe color of skin mucous membranes; observe for presence of hoarseness, stridor, and cough; monitor heart rate and regularity; observe behavior
2.
   a. assess respiratory status and detect any impending airway obstruction
   b. ease respiratory efforts
   c. prevent dehydration
   d. be prepared to assist with tracheostomy
   e. provide nutrition
   f. reduce parental anxiety
3. to liquefy respiratory secretions and decrease the edema of the respiratory tract

Section IV D

1. Respiratory syncytial virus (RSV) accounts for largest percentage
2. *Mycoplasma pneumoniae*
3. *Pneumococcus, Streptococcus, Staphylococcus*
4. Fever, slight cough, and prostration
5. Fever, chills, headache, malaise, anorexia, myalgia, rhinitis, sore throat, dry hacking cough; mucopurulent or blood-streaked sputum
6. poor feeding, fever, tachypnea, cough, chills, rales, rhonchi, pleural effusion and pain; pain may be referred to abdomen.
7. Symptomatic
8. Symptomatic
9. Antimicrobial therapy directed at causative organism, pneumococcal vaccine

Section IV E

1.
   a. Do not allow access to small items that might be placed in mouth. Balloons are another hazard.
   b. Refrain from use of talcum powder, oily nose drops, oil-based vitamin preparations. Position on the right side or abdomen after feedings.

Section IV F

1. the history of eczema as a baby; maternal history of hayfever; paternal history of asthma during childhood
2. hacking, nonproductive cough, shortness of breath
3. productive cough; audible wheezing upon expiration; restlessness and apprehension; sweating; use of accessory muscles; rapid respirations; upright position with hunched shoulders
4.
   a. relief of bronchospasm
   b. tachycardia, increased blood pressure, pallor, weakness, tremors, and nausea
5. skin color for cyanosis; character of respirations; presence of retractions; nasal flaring; breath sounds; and mental status
6. Child sweats profusely, remains sitting upright, and refuses to lie down. A child who suddenly becomes agitated or suddenly becomes quiet may be seriously hypoxic.
7.
   a. Eliminate or avoid proven or suspicious irritants and allergens
   b. Relieve bronchospasm
   c. Maintain optimum health
   d. Prevent complications
   e. Promote normal activities
   f. Support and educate child and family regarding the disease and its management

Section IV G

1.
   a. potential for infection related to impaired body defenses
   b. altered nutrition: less than body requirements related to inability to digest nutrients
   c. activity intolerance related to imbalance between oxygen supply and demand
   d. ineffective airway clearance related to secretion of thick tenacious mucus
   e. ineffective breathing pattern related to tracheobronchial obstruction
   f. impaired gas exchange related to airway obstruction
   g. altered growth and development related to inadequate digestion of nutrients
   h. altered family process related to situational crisis
   i. anticipatory grieving related to perceived potential loss of child
   j. impaired social interaction related to hospitalization, home confinement, fatigue

2. Dennis manages secretions with minimum distress.

3.
  a. obstruction of bronchioles and bronchi with abnormally thick mucus
  b. lack of trypsin, amylase, and lipase causes large amounts of undigested food which are excreted
  c. because so little food is absorbed from intestine, the child tries to compensate
  d. appetite can't compensate for fecal wastage
  e. inability to absorb fat-soluble vitamins

4.
  a. postural drainage technique
  b. breathing exercises
  c. aerosol therapy

Section IV H

1. tuberculin test
2.
  a. two or more drugs are usually required
  b. drugs must be continued for a long time, so compliance is a concern

Chapter 23

Question   Answer

Section III

1. the total output of fluid exceeds the total intake.
2. c
3. T
4. c
5. It is defined as a noticeable or sudden increase in the number of stools, a reduction in their consistency with increase in fluid content, and as stools that are green in color.
6. F
7. d
8. polymorphonuclear leukocytes ("polys")
9. meeting ongoing daily physiologic losses; replacing previous deficits; and replacing ongoing abnormal losses.
10. fecal-oral route; contaminated food
11. F
12. carbohydrate malabsorption
13. T
14. reduced severity and duration of illness
15. shigella
16. Giardia; cryptosporidium
17. Environmental change
18. autonomic parasympathetic ganglion cells

19. absence of propulsive movement (peristalsis)
20. rectal biopsy
21. surgical correction
22. transfer of gastric contents into the esophagus
23.
  a. flat prone
  b. head-elevated prone
24.
  a. right lower quadrant abdominal pain
  b. fever
  c. rigid abdomen
  d. decreased or absent bowel sounds
  e. vomiting
  f. constipation or diarrhea may be present
  g. anorexia
  h. tachycardia, rapid shallow breathing
  i. pallor
  j. lethargy
  k. irritability
  l. stooped posture
25. McBurney's point; anterosuperior iliac crest and the umbilicus
26. F
27. outpouching of the ileum
28. the diverticulum contains gastric mucosa, which produces hydrochloric acid, which irritates the bowel and erodes the intestinal surface
29. history
30. surgery
31. Ulcerative colitis
32. sulfasalazine
33. ulcerative colitis
34. pain - burning or gnawing sensation in epigastrium related to fasting state; melena; hematemesis; waking at night crying with pain; obstruction.
35.
  a. relieve discomfort
  b. promote healing
  c. prevent complications
  d. prevent recurrence
36.
  a. Hepatitis A virus (HAV)
  b. Hepatitis B virus (HBV)
  c. Hepatitis C virus (HCV, or classic non-A non-B)
  d. Hepatitis D virus (HDV, delta agent)
  e. Hepatitis E virus (epidemic non-A non-B)
37.
  a. oral, fecal
  b. parenteral
  c. usually rapid acute
  d. more insidious
  e. present after one attack, no crossover to Type B
  f. present after one attack

38. hepatitis B surface antigen

39.
- a. T
- b. F
- c. F
- d. F
- e. T

40. cell injury; tissue repair; regeneration; irreversible

41. progressive cirrhosis, death

42. defective speech

43. feeding

44.
- a. excessive salivation and drooling
- b. coughing, choking, cyanosis
- c. apnea
- d. increased respiratory distress following feeding
- e. abdominal distention

45. coughing; choking; cyanosis

46. protrusion of a portion of an organ or organs through the abdominal wall.

47. incarcerated

48. projectile

49. pyloromyotomy

50. an invagination or telescoping of one portion of the intestine into another

51. red, currant-jelly-like

52. barium enema

53. Malabsorption syndrome

54. intestinal mucosal transport system

55.
- a. impaired fat absorption
- b. impaired absorption of nutrients
- c. behavioral changes
- d. celiac crisis

56. celiac crisis

57.
- a. to preserve as much length of bowel as possible during surgery
- b. to maintain the child's nutritional status until adaptation to the altered bowel takes place
- c. to stimulate the adaptation process of the bowel

Section IV A

1.
- a. accurate history of bowel habits
- b. diet and events that may be associated with the onset of constipation
- c. drugs or other substances that the child may be taking
- d. consistency, color, frequency, and other characteristics of the stool

Section IV B

1.
- a. to help the parents adjust to a congenital defect in their child
- b. to foster infant-parent bonding
- c. to prepare them for the medical-surgical intervention
- d. to assist them in colostomy care after discharge

2.
- a. creation of temporary colostomy
- b. surgical correction—"pulling through"
- c. closure of colostomy

Section IV C

1. Position infant in prone position with head elevated at 30-degree angle for 24 hours/day. Maintain position with a body harness, or leave flat-prone.

2.
- a. identifying children with symptoms of GER
- b. helping parents with positioning and feeding at home
- c. providing reassurance to parents regarding the benign nature of the condition
- d. providing care if child requires surgical repair

Section IV D

1. degree of change in his behavior

2.
- a. listen for return of bowel sounds
- b. observe for passage of stool

Section IV E

1. chronic inflammatory reaction involving mucosa and submucosa of large intestine; mucosa becomes hyperemic and edematous with formation of patchy granulations over intestinal surface that bleed easily and lead to development of superficial ulcerations

2. affects the terminal ileum and involves all layers of bowel wall; acute edema and inflammation progress to keep ulcerations often associated with fissure formations leading to obstruction

3. common

4. uncommon

5. often severe

6. moderate to absent

7. less frequent

8. common

9. mild or moderate
10. can be severe
11. moderate
12. severe
13. usually mild
14. often marked

Section IV F

1.
    a. severity of hepatitis
    b. rigidity of medical regimen
    c. factors influencing control and transmission of the disease
2.
    a. a well-balanced diet and a realistic schedule of rest and activity adjusted to the child's condition

Section IV G

1. the feeding process is often time consuming and very difficult. Clefts of the lip or palate reduce the infant's ability to suck, which interferes with compression of the areola and usually renders both breast- and bottle-feeding difficult.
2.
    a. prevent injury to operative site
    b. provide nutrition
    c. prevent complications
    d. support child and family
3. Operative site remains undamaged

Section IV H

1.
    a. give small frequent feedings
    b. bubble before and frequently during feedings
    c. position in high Fowler's and slightly on right side after feedings
    d. handle minimally and gently after feedings
2. This position facilitates the passage of formula through the pylorus and prevents vomiting from occurring.
3. anxiety, related to separation from accustomed routine and environment
4. You would have the parents demonstrate the infant's care in the hospital to see whether they provide optimum care.

Section IV I

1.
    a. (1) Explain diagnosis: (2) encourage parents to room-in; (3) explain procedures and equipment; and (4) support parents through this sudden emergency.

    b. (1) Explain and demonstrate why this is being performed; (2) assure the parents that you will accompany Jason to x-ray and support the child through the procedure.

Section IV J

1.
    a. explaining why she must be NPO for 4 to 8 hours before the procedure
    b. explaining why a tube is passed through the mouth
    c. supporting Patricia during the test
2. foods containing wheat, rye, barley and oats; processed foods containing hydrolyzed vegetable protein

Chapter 24

Question   **Answer**

Section III

1. a
2. foramen ovale; ductus arteriosus
3. F
4. acyanotic; cyanotic
5. left; right
6. right; left
7.
    a. 1
    b. 2
    c. 1, 7
    d. 3
    e. 5
    f. 4
    g. 2
    h. 7
    i. 6
    j. 4
8. ventricular septal defect; atrial septal defect; patent ductus arteriosus; coarctation of aorta; pulmonic stenosis; aortic stenosis
9. the inability of the heart to pump an adequate amount of blood to the systemic circulation to meet the body's metabolic demands
10. increased blood volume and pressure
11.
    a. right-sided failure
    b. left-sided failure
12. tachycardia
13. tachypnea, dyspnea, retractions, flaring nares, exercise intolerance, orthopnea, cough, hoarseness, cyanosis, wheezing, grunting.

14. hepatomegaly; edema; weight gain
15.
   a. improve cardiac function
   b. remove accumulated fluid and sodium
   c. decrease cardiac demands
   d. improve tissue oxygenation and decrease oxygen consumption
16.
   a. allow period of grief
   b. accept initial shock and disbelief
   c. repeat information as often as necessary
   d. foster parent-child attachment
   e. introduce parents to other families who have similarly affected child
17. *Streptococcus viridans*
18. mitral valve
19. group A streptococcal
20. Jones; streptococcal; ASO
21.
   a. contain low concentrations of triglycerides, high levels of cholesterol, and moderate levels of protein.
   b. contain very low concentrations of triglycerides, relatively little cholesterol, and high levels of protein.
22.
   a. Bradydysrhythmias
   b. Tachydysrhythmias
   c. Conduction disturbances
23. recognition of an abnormal heartbeat, either in rate or rhythm
24. blood pressure
25. Surgery; hypertensive drug
26. Kawasaki disease; cardiovascular
27. temperature
28. aspirin and gamma globulin
29.
   a. hypotension
   b. tissue hypoxia
   c. metabolic acidosis
30.
   a. compensated
   b. uncompensated
   c. irreversible shock
31. F
32.
   a. ventilation
   b. fluid administration
   c. improvement of the pumping action of the heart
33. the interaction of an allergen and a patient who is hypersensitive.
34. flushing; urticaria; angioedema - noticed in eyelids, lips, tongue, hands, feet, and genitalia.
35. T

36.
   a. primary feature - rash
   b. arthritic effects
   c. gastrointestinal involvement
   d. renal involvement

Section IV A

1.
   a. level of understanding, especially cognitive skills
   b. past experiences
   c. understanding and perception of the situation
2.
   a. detects abnormalities in rate and rhythm
   b. detects cardiac hemorrhage from perforation or bleeding at the site of the initial catheterization
   c. detects vessel obstruction
   d. detects possible vessel obstruction

Section IV B

1.
   a. C
   b. X
   c. C
   d. C
   e. C
   f. X
   g. C
   h. C
   i. X
   j. C
2.
   a. maternal rubella; poor nutrition; diabetes; maternal age over 40 years; maternal alcoholism
   b. increased risk of congenital heart disease in a child who (1) has a sibling with a heart defect, (2) has a parent with congenital heart disease, (3) has a chromosomal aberration, or (4) is born with other noncardiac congenital anomalies
3. a loud, harsh, pansystolic murmur

Section IV C

1.
   a. improves cardiac functioning by such beneficial effects as increased cardiac output, decreased heart size, decreased venous pressure, and relief of edema
   b. remove accumulated fluid and sodium
2.
   a. count the apical pulse for one full minute

before administering digitalis, and withhold dose if pulse is lower than either 90-110 in infants or 70 in older children

b. calculate dosage accurately

c. use correct preparation of digitalis (use digoxin)

d. monitor serum potassium levels

3. Low potassium increases the cardiac effects of digitalis.

4. nausea, vomiting, anorexia, bradycardia, dysrhythmias

5.

a. administer digitalis; observe for signs of digitalis toxicity; institute teaching regarding drug administration at home; attach cardiac monitor

b. provide for optimum rest periods; conserve child's energy for feeding; minimize child's crying and stress; maintain child's body temperature

c. position in semi- to high-Fowler's position; carefully assess child's respiratory status; administer oxygen prn

d. administer diuretics as ordered; carefully monitor intake and output; monitor body weight; provide skin care; position frequently.

Section IV D

1.

a. 1, 3, 9

b. 1, 4

c. 1, 6

d. 2, 5, 7

e. 6, 8

Section IV E

1.

a. fluid volume deficit related to increased body temperature

b. sensory-perceptual alterations (visual) related to inflammation of the eyes

c. altered nutrition: less than body requirements, related to inadequate intake

d. potential impaired skin integrity related to irritation of edematous tissue and denuded skin

e. pain related to itchy rash

f. pain related to swelling in cervical region

2.

a. administer aspirin, teach the family signs of aspirin toxicity, monitor the temperature frequently, promote rest, give tepid sponge baths

b. encourage fluids, keep accurate intake and output records, take and record daily

weight, monitor temperature status, assess skin turgor, monitor urine specific gravity

c. administer aspirin as ordered, observe for signs of myocarditis and congestive heart failure, monitor vital signs frequently, observe for behavioral changes, teach parents the need for close follow-up care

Chapter 25

Question	Answer

Section III

1.

a. Red blood cell (RBC)

b. Hemoglobin (Hgb)

c. Hematocrit (Hct)

d. RBC indexes

e. RBC volume distribution

f. Reticulocyte count

g. White blood cell (WBC)

h. Differential WBC count

i. Absolute neutrophil count

j. Platelet count

k. Stained peripheral blood smear

2. reduction of red blood cells

3.

a. Etiology and physiology—the causes of erythrocyte and hemoglobin depletion

b. Morphology—the characteristic changes in red cell size, shape, color

4.

a. blood loss

b. increased destruction of RBCs

c. impaired or decreased rate of production

5.

a. 4

b. 7

c. 5

d. 9

e. 8

f. 6

g. 3

h. 2

i. 1

6.

a. average or mean volume of a single RBC

b. mean quantity of hemoglobin in a single RBC

c. mean concentration of hemoglobin in a single RBC

d. number of RBC/mm^3 of blood

e. amount of Hgb/100 ml of whole blood

f. percentage or volume of packed RBC to whole blood

g. percentage of reticulocytes to RBCs

h. number of WBC/mm^3 of blood

i. inspection and quantification of WBC types present in peripheral blood

j. number of platelets in blood

7. decrease in the oxygen-carrying capacity of the blood

8.
a. muscle weakness and easy fatigability; pale skin; pica

b. headache; dizziness, lightheadedness; irritability; slowed thought processes; decreased attention span; apathy and depression

c. increased heart rate, poor peripheral perfusion, skin moist and cool, low blood pressure and central venous pressure

9.
a. prepare child for diagnostic test and possible blood transfusion

b. decrease tissue oxygen needs

c. implement safety precautions

d. observe for complications

10. Iron

11. Children become anemic because they drink milk, a poor source of iron, almost to the exclusion of solid foods

12. vomiting, diarrhea, staining of teeth

13. prevention of nutritional anemia through education of family

14. tarry green color

15.
a. sickle cell trait–the heterozygous form of the disease (HbA + HbS, or HbSA)

b. sickle cell anemia–the homozygous form of the disease (HbS)

16. sickle-shaped

17. oxygenation; hemodilution

18.
a. increased blood viscosity

b. increased red blood cell destruction

19. infection

20.
a. vaso-occlusive crisis

b. sequestration crisis

c. aplastic crisis

d. hyperhemolytic crisis

21. Sickeldex

22. no

23. can depress bone marrow activity and further aggravate anemia

24. overwhelming infection

25. hemoglobin chain; Cooley anemia; compatible

26. red blood cells; anemia; life span; hemosiderin, hemosiderosis

27. Deferoxamine

28. A group of bleeding disorders in which there is a deficiency of one of the factors necessary for coagulation of blood

29. Classic hemophilia
a. factor VIII

b. factor IX

30. X-linked recessive disorder

31. joint cavities; hemarthrosis

32. intracranial hemorrhage

33. replacement of the missing factor

34. factor VIII concentrate

35.
a. excessive destruction of platelets

b. purpura (a discoloration caused by petechiae beneath the skin)

36. T

37. the initial white blood count; the patient's age at diagnosis; the histologic type of the disease; sex; karyotype analysis

38.
a. a low leukocyte count, but a greatly increased count of immature cells or "blasts"

b. cellular destruction in the bone marrow by infiltration and subsequent competition for metabolic elements

39. anemia; infection; bleeding tendencies; bone weakness and invasion of periosteum

40. fever, pallor; fatigue; hemorrhage; bone and joint pain; tendency to fracture

41. increased intracranial pressure

42. bone marrow aspiration; biopsy

43. remission induction; CNS preventive therapy and consolidation; maintenance

44. the central nervous system

45.
a. corticosteroids; vincristine; and L-asparaginase, with or without doxorubicin, daunomycin, and cytosine

b. methotrexate and cranial irradiation, cystosine arabinoside, L-asparaginase

c. combined drug regimens

46. Hodgkin disease originates in the lymphoid system and primarily involves the lymph nodes. It predictably metastasizes to non-nodal or extralymphatic sites, especially the spleen, liver, bone marrow, and lungs. Non-Hodgkin lymphoma in children is strikingly different from Hodgkin disease. The disease is usually diffuse, rather than nodular; the cell type is either undifferentiated or poorly differentiated; dissemination occurs early, more often than in Hodgkin disease, and rapidly; mediastinal involvement and invasion of meninges are common.

47. enlargement of lymph nodes
48. radiation; chemotherapy
49. direct contact; intimate sexual contact
50. perinatal transmission
51. preventing transmission of the virus
52.

    a. HIV
    b. no cure; primarily supportive; prevention and management of the opportunistic infections, some use of AZT
    c. fatal

53. a defect characterized by absence of both humoral and cell-mediated immunity
54. bone-marrow transplant
55.

    a. thrombocytopenia
    b. eczema
    c. immunodeficiency of selective functions of B- and T-lymphocytes.

56.

    a. hemolytic reactions
    b. febrile reactions
    c. allergic reactions
    d. circulatory overload
    e. air emboli
    f. hypothermia
    g. electrolyte disturbances

57.

    a. allogeneic
    b. autologous
    c. syngeneic

Section IV A

1.

    a. explaining the significance of each test
    b. physically being with the child during the procedure
    c. allowing the child to play with the equipment on a doll and/or participate in the actual procedure

2.

    a. Anxiety/fear related to diagnostic procedures/transfusion
    b. Activity intolerance related to generalized weakness, diminished oxygen delivery to tissues

Section IV B

1.

    a. avoid strenuous physical activity; avoid emotional stress; avoid environments of low oxygen concentration; avoid known sources of infection
    b. calculate the child's daily fluid requirements; assess the child's actual fluid con-

sumption; encourage fluids; assess signs of dehydration; teach parents how to assess fluid status; monitor output

2.

    a. Pain related to tissue ischemia
    b. Altered tissue perfusion related to impaired arterial blood flow

3. child plays and rests quietly and engages in activities appropriate to capabilities

Section IV C

1. headache; slurred speech; loss of consciousness; black tarry stools
2.

    a. Apply pressure to area of bleeding for 10 to 15 minutes—to allow clot formation.
    b. Immobilize and elevate area above the level of the heart—to decrease blood flow.
    c. Apply cold—to promote vasoconstriction.

Section IV D

1.

    a. prevent hemorrhage
    b. prevent hemorrhagic cystitis
    c. prevent or reduce the effects of anemia

2.

    a. provide meticulous skin care
    b. change position frequently
    c. encourage adequate calorie-protein intake

Section IV E

1.

    a. wear gloves
    b. careful handwashing
    c. wear gowns
    d. wear masks and eye protection
    e. precaution with needles and syringes
    f. precaution with trash and linen

2.

    a. Potential for infection related to impaired body defenses, presence of infective organisms
    b. Impaired social interaction
    c. Altered sexuality pattern
    d. Altered family processes related to having a child with a dreaded and life-threatening disease

Chapter 26

Question   Answer

Section III

1. urinary stasis
2. F
3.
    a. eliminate infection
    b. detect and correct functional or anatomic abnormalities
    c. prevent recurrence
    d. preserve renal function
4.
    a. congenital or acquired
    b. unilateral or bilateral
    c. complete or incomplete
    d. acute or chronic
5. the collection of urine in the renal pelvis to the point of cyst formation from the distention
6. b
7. c
8. Corticosteroids
9. a
10.
    a. 2
    b. 2
    c. 1
    d. 2
    e. 1
11.
    a. history of a sore throat and/or skin infection
    b. urine analysis
    c. ASO titer
    d. elevated AHase and ADNase-B titers and ANADase titers
    e. decreased serum complement levels
    f. CBC
    g. throat culture
12. F
13. T
14. proximal tubules; glomeruli
15. T
16. Hemolytic uremic syndrome
17. the lining of the small glomerular arterioles
18.
    a. vomiting
    b. pallor
    c. irritability
    d. lethargy
    e. anuria or oliguria
    f. hemorrhagic manifestations
    g. central nervous system involvement
    h. signs of acute heart failure
19. the damage to the red blood cells in the arterioles and the subsequent hemolysis
20. c
21. oliguria
22. F
23.
    a. treating the underlying cause
    b. management of the complications of renal failure
    c. provision of supportive therapy
24. hyperkalemia; hypertension
25. F
26. the process of separating colloids and crystalline substances in solution by the difference in their rate of diffusion through a semipermeable membrane.
27.
    a. peritoneal dialysis
    b. hemodialysis
    c. hemofiltration
28. renal transplantation

Section IV A

1.
    a. fever
    b. frequent urination
    c. poor feeding
    d. failure to gain weight
    e. dehydration
2. The incidence of UTI in males is greater in infancy. This is usually the result of some sort of obstruction that results in urinary stasis. Also, the presence of a large or greater than normal output is suggestive of obstructive uropathy.
3. prevention
4.
    a. injury: potential for, related to presence of infected organism and anatomic abnormality
    b. altered family process related to situational crisis
5.
    a. collection of specimen
    b. prepare Barry's parents for diagnostic procedure
    c. administer antimicrobials as ordered
    d. monitor vital signs
    e. monitor urine output
    f. teach Barry's parents how to prevent recurrences
    g. teach Barry's parents how to perform his home care
6. You would observe Barry's parents caring for him to see if they are putting the diaper on too tight and if they are cleaning his genitals well.

Section IV B

1. fluid volume deficit related to protein loss and fluid excess
2. Prevent and control acute infection
3.
   a. offer high-protein, high-carbohydrate diet
   b. enlist the aid of the child and parents in formulation of diet
   c. provide a cheerful, relaxed environment
   d. provide special and preferred foods
   e. serve foods in an attractive manner
   f. serve small quantities
4. The presence of edema may predispose the child to skin breakdown and may make routine care more difficult. Also, because of low protein levels, the child is predisposed to infection and breakdown.
5.
   a. maintaining bed rest
   b. balance rest and activity
   c. plan and provide quiet activities
   d. instruct the child to rest when fatigued
6. Teach the family urine testing, administration of medications, signs of relapse, side effects of drugs, and prevention of infection.
7. The parents are able to test the urine and administer the medications correctly. They understand your instructions concerning prevention of infection, signs of relapse, and side effects of drugs.

Section IV C

1. The nurse should have instructed Tina's mother to continue the antibiotics for the total prescribed time, even if Tina should feel better.
2. prevent fluid accumulation
3.
   a. encourage her parents to visit
   b. spend time with the child
   c. provide an opportunity to socialize with noninfected children
   d. provide appropriate play activities
4.
   a. monitor fluid balance
   b. weigh child daily
   c. measure intake and output
   d. measure specific gravity of urine
   e. observe for signs of dehydration and overload
   f. monitor vital signs
5. Protein is restricted in children with acute renal failure to prevent the accumulation of nitrogenous wastes.
6. The family members demonstrate an understanding of the information presented and express their feelings and concerns.

Section IV D

1. anorexia, irritability, lethargy, pallor, hemorrhagic manifestations, oliguria or anuria, central nervous system manifestations, signs of heart failure
2. potential for infection related to diminished body defenses
3.
   a. prevent dietary deficiencies
   b. prevent retention of waste products
4.
   a. assess home situation
   b. teach the family home care
   c. help family acquire needed drugs and equipment
   d. assist family in problem solving
   e. assist family in diet planning
   f. prepare the child and family for home peritoneal dialysis
   g. maintain periodic contact
5.
   a. monitor fluid intake
   b. provide low sodium diet
   c. administer diuretics
   d. administer antihypertensive medications
6.
   a. engage in activities appropriate for her age
   b. discuss her feelings and concerns
   c. comply with medication, diet, and dialysis regimen

Section IV E

1.
   a. Keep explanations simple, and repeat them often.
   b. The nurse should be present during physician-parent conferences to answer questions that arise after the conference.
2.
   a. monitor bowel movements
   b. auscultate for bowel sounds
   c. monitor for abdominal distention or vomiting

Chapter 27

Question   Answer

Section III

1.
   a. family history
   b. health history
   c. physical evaluation of infants

2.

    a. irritability; high-pitched cry; cries when held or rocked; bulging fontanels; separated cranial sutures; increased occipital frontal circumference; change in feeding patterns

    b. headache; nausea; vomiting; diplopia; drowsiness; diminished physical activity and motor performance; fatigue; memory loss; seizures

3. lowered level of consciousness; decreased motor response to painful stimuli; alterations in pupil size and reactivity; sometimes decerebrate or decorticate posturing; Cheyne-Stokes respiration; and papilledema.

4.

    a. observation of spontaneous and elicited reflex responses

    b. observation of the development of increasingly complex locomotor and fine motor skills

    c. eliciting of progressively more sophisticated communicative and adaptive behaviors

    d. observing for the presence of a primitive reflex beyond the time it would normally disappear

5. history; physical examination

6. an estimation of the level of development

7.

    a. alertness—an aroused or waking state that includes the ability to respond to stimuli

    b. cognitive power—the ability to process stimuli and produce verbal and motor responses

8. the patient's responses to his environment

9. sleep, confusion, delirium, pseudowakeful states, and comatose states

10.

    a. eye opening

    b. verbal response

    c. motor response

11. establish an accurate, objective baseline of neurologic function

12. vital signs, skin, eyes, motor function and posturing, and reflexes

13. neurosurgical emergency

14.

    a. lumbar puncture

    b. subdural tap

    c. electroencephalogram (EEG)

    d. video EEG

    e. computerized tomography

    f. transillumination

    g. brain scan

    h. echoencephalography

    i. MRI and NMR

    j. positron emission

    k. ultrasonography

    l. angiography

    m. radiography

15. patent airway

16.

    a. concussion—a transient and reversible neuronal dysfunction with instantaneous loss of awareness and responsiveness for minutes or hours.

    b. contusion and laceration—visible bruising and tearing of cerebral tissue

    c. fracture—a break in the skull that is linear, depressed, compound, basilar, and diastolic

17.

    a. hemorrhage

    b. infection

    c. edema

    d. herniation through the tentorium

18. Accumulation of blood between the skull and cerebral surfaces is dangerous because it can compress the underlying brain and produce effects that can be rapidly fatal or insidiously progressive.

19. Nonspecific complaints such as irritability; headache; vomiting.

20. hematoma

21. between the dura and the cerebrum; cortical veins

22. cerebral edema

23. Intracranial pressure exceeds arterial pressure and fatal anoxia ensues and/or the pressure causes herniation of a portion of the brain over the edge of the tentorium, compressing the brainstem and occluding the posterior cerebral arteries.

24. computed tomography

25. assessment of the child's LOC

26. the length of submersion, the physiologic response of the victim, and the development and degree of immersion hypothermia

27.

    a. hypoxia and asphyxiation

    b. aspiration

    c. hypothermia

28. prevented

29. medulloblastoma, cerebellar astrocytoma, brainstem glioma, ependymomas, and gliomas.

30. because their sutures are still open and an increase in the size of the head is not readily detected.

31. CAT scan

32. removal

33. infectious process

34. cerebral edema

35. because it increases intracranial pressure and the risk of hemorrhage.

36. adrenal gland or retroperitoneal sympathetic chain

37. primary site; areas of metastasis

38. by analyzing the breakdown products that are normally excreted in the urine, namely vanillylmandelic acid (VMA)
39.
   a. surgery
   b. radiotherapy
   c. chemotherapy
40. invasiveness
41.
   a. *Hemophilus influenzae* (type B)
   b. *Streptococcus pneumoniae*
   c. *Neisseria meningitidis* (Meningococcus)
42. Meningococcal meningitis is readily transmitted by droplet infection from nasopharyngeal secretions.
43. examination of the cerebrospinal fluid by lumbar puncture
44.
   a. F
   b. F
   c. F
45. symptomatic
46.
   a. direct invasion of the central nervous system
   b. postinfectious involvement of the central nervous system after a viral disease
47. influenza; varicella
48. aspirin
49. unexplained neurodevelopmental regression and focal seizures in a child with AIDS
50.
   a. the inactivated rabies vaccines
   b. the globulins, which contain preformed antibodies
51. initiated by a group of hyperexcitable cells referred to as the epileptogenic focus. When neuronal excitation from the epileptogenic focus spreads to the brain stem, a generalized seizure develops.
52. generalized seizures and partial seizures
53. a period of altered behavior for which the individual is amnesic and during which he is unable to respond to his environment. There is no loss of consciousness during attack.
54. electroencephalogram
55.
   a. control the seizures or reduce their frequency
   b. discover and correct the cause of seizures
   c. who has recurrent seizures to live as normal a life as possible
56. The action of anticonvulsive drugs is to raise the threshold of excitability and prevent seizures
57. The drug should be reduced gradually over 1 to 2 weeks.
58. The drugs are monitored by taking frequent serum blood levels.
59. grand mal

60. absence seizure, petit mal
61. a continuous seizure that lasts more than 30 minutes or as serial seizures from which the child does not regain a premorbid level of consciousness.
62. Siderails raised when child is sleeping; siderails padded; waterproof mattress/pad on bed/crib; appropriate precautions during potentially hazardous activities; have child carry or wear medical identification; alert other caregivers to need for any special precautions.
63. transient disorders of children that occur in association with a fever.
64. normal
65. Hydrocephalus
66.
   a. impaired absorption of CSF within the subarachnoid space
   b. obstruction to the flow of CSF within the ventricles
67.
   a. abnormally rapid head growth
   b. bulging fontanels
   c. dilated scalp veins
   d. separated sutures
   e. Macewen sign on percussion
   f. thinning of skull bones
   g. frontal enlargement or "bossing"
   h. depressed eyes - "setting sun" sign
   i. sluggish pupils with unequal response to light
68. T
69. CAT scan; MRI

Section IV A

1. alteration in neurologic status related to increased intracranial pressure
2. delirium

Section IV B

1.
   a. maintain patent airway
   b. prevent intracranial pressure (ICP)
   c. prevent cerebral hypoxia
   d. prevent cerebral edema
   e. prevent seizures
   f. prevent or control hyperthermia
   g. prevent respiratory infection
   h. prevent corneal irritation
   i. prevent drying of mucous membranes
   j. protect from physical injury
   k. maintain limb flexibility and functions
   l. maintain skin integrity
   m. ensure adequate fluid intake
   n. ensure adequate nutritional intake

o. provide hygienic care

p. provide toileting and ensure adequate elimination

q. provide sensory stimulation

r. relieve discomfort

s. support family

t. assist in child placement, if indicated

2. vital signs, pupillary reactions, level of consciousness

3.

    a. elevate head of bed 15 to 30 degrees

    b. avoid positions or activities that increase ICP

    c. prevent constipation

    d. provide quiet environment and decrease stress

    e. Administer paralyzing agents if prescribed

4. to prevent pressure on prominent areas of the body

Section IV C

1. vital signs, neurologic signs, and level of consciousness

2. assure parent that everything possible is being done to treat the child; repeat message often

Section IV D

1. Clinical manifestations include fever, vomiting, marked irritability, seizures, a high-pitched cry and a bulging fontanel. Nuchal rigidity may or may not be present. Brudzinski and Kernig signs are not usually used in making the diagnosis since they are difficult to evaluate in children in this age group.

2.

    a. isolation

    b. initiation of antimicrobial therapy

    c. maintenance of optimum hydration

    d. maintenance of ventilation

    e. reduction of increased ICP

    f. management of bacterial shock

    g. control of seizures

    h. control of extremes of temperature

    i. correction of anemia

    j. treatment of complications

Section IV E

1.

    a. description of child's behavior before and during a seizure

    b. the age of onset of first seizure

    c. the usual time at which the seizure occurs

    d. any factors that may have precipitated the seizure

    e. any sensory phenomena that the child can describe

    f. duration and progression of the seizure

    g. postictal feelings and behavior

2.

    a. do not attempt to restrain child or use force

    b. remove objects

    c. do not move or forcefully restrain her

    d. do not force object between clenched teeth

    e. protect her from injury on siderails

    f. allow seizures to end without interference

3.

    a. Help the family to establish time of administration of medication to coincide with the family routine.

    b. The tablet form of the drug is the preferred form; crush and administer in syrup or jelly.

    c. Emphasize that the medication must be continued for as long as required.

    d. Explain the need for adequate vitamin D and folic acid.

    e. Teach what side effects may occur.

    f. Explain why periodic blood studies are necessary.

    g. Explain the degree to which activities are restricted.

Section IV F

1. a

2.

    a. High risk for infection related to presence of mechanical drainage system

    b. High risk from impaired skin integrity related to pressure areas, paralysis, relaxed anal sphincter

    c. Altered family processes related to situational crisis

3. family discusses their feelings and concerns regarding the child's condition

Chapter 28

Question   **Answer**

Section III

1. hypophysis; master gland

2. idiopathic factors

3. short stature

4. growth hormone

5.

    a. surgical removal or irradiation of tumor

    b. replacement of growth hormone

6. overgrowth of long bones; overgrowth in transverse direction; acromegaly
7. increasing intracranial pressure
8. early identification of children with inappropriate growth rates
9. diabetes insipidus; diuresis
10. polyuria; polydipsia
11. vasopressin
12. syndrome of inappropriate secretion of antidiuretic hormone; fluid retention; hypotonicity
13. thyroid
14. to regulate the basal metabolic rate
15. an enlargement or hypertrophy of the thyroid gland; iodine
16. thyroid gland
17. acute onset: severe irritability and restlessness; vomiting; diarrhea; hyperthermia; hypertension; severe tachycardia; prostration; may progress to delirium, coma, death
18. hypoparathyroidism
19. calcium; phosphate
20. Hyperparathyroidism
21.
  a. 1
  b. 2
  c. 2
  d. 1
  e. 1
22.
  a. 1
  b. 2
23. iatrogenic Cushing syndrome
24. moon
25. sexual
26. genotype
27. adrenogenital syndrome
28. familial; dominant
29. increased production of catecholamines
30.
  a. glucagon–stimulates liver to release stored glucose
  b. insulin–facilitates entrance of glucose into the cells for metabolism
  c. somatostatin–regulates release of insulin and glucagon
31. IDDM; NIDDM; MODY
32.
  a. less than 20 years
  b. over 40 years
  c. 45%–60% develop
  d. 100% develop
  e. polyphagia, polyuria, polydipsia
  f. overweight, fatigue, frequent infections
  g. yes
  h. infrequent
33.
  a. glucose is unable to enter cells, causing hyperglycemia

  b. glucose accumulates in bloodstream causing an osmotic gradient to occur, which results in fluid moving from the intracellular to the extracellular space
  c. fluid is filtered through the glomerulus into the renal tubule; the renal tubule reabsorbs the glucose and most of the water in the filtrate; when glucose concentrate exceeds the threshold, the glucose is excreted in the urine
  d. water is also excreted as part of the osmotic diversion
  e. urinary fluid losses cause the individual to experience thirst
  f. because glucose is unable to enter the cells, the body burns fat for energy but also uses protein
  g. the liver metabolizes protein and converts it to glucose for energy use
  h. because the body cannot use glucose, and fat and protein stores are depleted, the patient experiences hunger and increased food intake
  i. when fats are metabolized, they are broken down into fatty acids and ketone bodies; the ketone bodies are excreted in the urine and in the lungs
  j. the production of ketone bodies, which are organic acids, and the dehydration that results from the osmotic diuresis, lead to a metabolic acidosis
34.
  a. microvascular changes
    1) nephropathy
    2) retinopathy
    3) neuropathy
35. polyphagia, polydipsia, polyuria
36. glucose oxidase tapes; clinitest tablets
37. F
38. Insulin pumps
39. Home blood glucose monitoring
40. lowers
41. Glucagon
42. a physiologic reflex response to a decreased blood glucose level which results in release of stress hormones (epinephrine, growth hormone, and corticosteroids) and a rebound hyperglycemia
43.
  a. rapid assessment
  b. adequate insulin to reduce the elevated blood glucose
  c. fluids to overcome dehydration
  d. electrolyte replacement, especially potassium
44. potassium
45.
  a. rapid
  b. gradual

c. too much insulin; increased exercise with no increase in food intake; diminished food intake; gastroenteritis

d. too little insulin; improper diet; reduced exercise with no reduction in food; emotional stress; physical stress; drugs; illness

e. lability of mood; difficulty concentrating; shaky feeling; pallor; tremors; tachycardia, shallow respirations

f. increased thirst; signs of dehydration; acetone breath; rapid and deep respirations; weak pulse; diminished reflexes; dulled sensorium

g. shock; coma; death

h. acidosis; coma; death

i. glucose negative; acetone negative

j. glucose positive; acetone positive

k. decreased: 60 mg per 100 ml, or less

l. increased: 250 mg per 100 ml, or more

46. to enhance absorption

47. sugar

48. adolescent

Section IV A

1.
  a. short stature but proportional height and weight
  b. appear well-nourished
  c. retarded bone age proportional to height age
  d. premature aging
  e. tend to be relatively inactive and shun aggressive sports
  f. eruption of permanent teeth delayed
  g. teeth overcrowded and malpositioned
  h. sexual development delayed but normal

2.
  a. overgrowth of long bones; reaches height of 8 feet
  b. rapid and increased development of muscles and viscera
  c. weight is increased but is in proportion to height
  d. proportional enlargement of head circumference

3.
  a. polyuria
  b. polydipsia
  c. irritability
  d. dehydration signs

4. cessation or retardation of growth in an infant whose growth has previously been normal

5. early identification of children with hypothyroidism

6.
  a. institute seizure precautions
  b. institute safety precautions
  c. reduce environmental stimuli
  d. observe for signs of laryngospasm

Section IV B

1. to monitor the hyperpyrexia and shocklike state

2. Overdosage can precipitate complications.

3. cardiac irregularities, poor muscle control, and inappropriate serum electrolyte levels

Section IV C

1. immediate recognition of ambiguous genitalia in the newborn

2. to suppress the abnormally high secretion of adrenocorticotropic hormone

Section IV D

1.
  a.
    1) rapid assessment
    2) adequate insulin to reduce the elevated blood glucose
    3) fluids to overcome dehydration
    4) electrolyte replacement
  b. child exhibits adequate hydration

2. blood glucose monitoring

3. ensure day-to-day consistency in total calorie, protein, fat, and carbohydrate

4.
  a. irritability, shaky feeling, sweating, pallor, tremors, tachycardia, shallow respirations
  b. Give child simple sugar or glucagon

5.
  a. educate the child and family about the disease, assessment techniques, and therapy
  b. prevent ill effects from complications of diabetes
  c. promote a positive self-image in the child
  d. provide support to child and family

6. Child takes responsibility for management of disease commensurate with age and capabilities

Section IV E

1.
  a. Child and family will understand nature of diabetes.
  b. Child and family will understand principles of meal planning.
  c. Child and family will understand insulin medication.
  d. Child and family will be able to demonstrate an appropriate injection procedure.
  e. Child and family will be able to demonstrate appropriate testing of urine.
  f. Child and family will be able to monitor blood glucose level.

g. Child and family will be able to identify signs of hyperglycemia and hypoglycemia.

h. Appropriate exercise program will be planned.

i. Child and family will demonstrate accurate method of record keeping.

j. Child and family will emphasize importance of personal hygiene.

k. Child and family will demonstrate proper use of insulin pump.

l. Child will wear emergency identification.

Chapter 29

Question   Answer

Section III

1. T
2.
   a. protection
   b. impermeability
   c. heat regulation
   d. sensation
3.
   a. contact with injurious agents such as infectious organisms, toxic chemicals, and physical trauma
   b. hereditary factors
   c. a systemic disease of which the lesions are a cutaneous manifestation or some external factor that produces a reaction in the skin.
4.
   a. 4
   b. 2
   c. 1
   d. 5
   e. 3
5. structural or physiologic disruptions of the integument that call for normal or abnormal tissue repair responses.
6.
   a. partial thickness
   b. full thickness
   c. complex wounds that include muscle and/or bone
7.
   a. inflammation
   b. fibroplasia
   c. contraction
   d. scar maturation
8. normal saline
9.
   a. prevent further damage

b. eliminate the cause of the damage
c. prevent complications
d. provide relief from discomfort while tissues undergo healing

10. provide a moist healing environment; protect the wound from infection and trauma; provide compression in the event of anticipated bleeding or swelling; apply medication; absorb drainage; debride necrotic tissue; and reduce pain and tenderness

11.
   a. polyurethane films
   b. hydrocolloids
   c. hydrogel sheets

12. c

13. increased erythema; edema; purulent exudate; pain; increased temperature.

14.
   a. prevent secondary damage to the lesion
   b. promote wound healing
   c. relieve discomfort
   d. education and support the child and family

15. pruritus

16. cool the skin by evaporation, relieve itching and inflammation, and cleanse the area by loosening and removing crusts and debris

17. oatmeal; mineral oil

18. F

19.
   a. to prevent the spread of infection
   b. to prevent complications

20.
   a. administering parenteral antibiotics
   b. applying compresses
   c. maintaining the intravenous infusion

21.
   a. with inflammation and vesiculation
   b. by proliferating to form growths

22. griseofulvin; ketoconazole selenium sulfide shampoos

23. an inflammatory reaction of the skin to chemical substances, natural or synthetic, that evoke a hypersensitivity response or to those agents that cause direct irritation

24. prevent further exposure of the skin to the offending substance

25. F

26. d

27. Further doses of the medication should be withheld and the rash reported to the attending physician.

28. scabies; pediculosis capitis

29.
   a. interdigital surfaces
   b. axillary-cubital area
   c. popliteal folds
   d. inguinal region

30. lindane (Kwell)
31. b
32. epinephrine
33. T
34. urine, feces, soaps, detergents, ointments, and friction
35.
   a. minimize skin wetness
   b. allow the skin to maintain its normal acidic pH
   c. minimize the interaction of urine and feces
36.
   a. 2
   b. 1
   c. 3
37.
   a. relieve pruritus
   b. hydrate the skin
   c. reduce the inflammation
   d. prevent or control secondary infection
38. a chronic, recurrent, inflammatory reaction of the skin
39. acne vulgaris
40. b
41. benzoyl peroxide; tretinoin (retinoic acid)
42.
   a. percentage of the body burned
   b. depth of the injury
   c. location of the burn
43. d
44. b
45. Anemia is caused by direct heat destruction of red blood cells, hemolysis of injured red cells, and trapping of red cells in the microvascular thrombi of damaged cells.
46. hypoxia
47.
   a. stop the burning process
   b. begin emergency procedures
   c. cover the wound
   d. transport the child to medical aid
   e. provide reassurance
48.
   a. to establish and maintain an adequate airway
   b. to establish a lifeline for fluid resuscitation
   c. to care for the burn wound
49.
   a. compensate for water and sodium lost to traumatized areas and interstitial spaces
   b. replenish sodium deficits
   c. restore plasma volume
   d. obtain adequate perfusion
   e. correct acidosis
   f. improve renal function
50. the infection rate and threat of sepsis

51.
   a. a topical antimicrobial ointment is applied directly to the wound surface, but the wound is left uncovered
   b. an ointment is applied directly to the wound or impregnated into thin gauze that is applied to the wound; a stretched gauze net secures the area
52. tissues obtained from human species, living or dead, usually cadavers, that are free from disease
53.
   a. prevent acute complications
   b. relieve pain
   c. facilitate wound healing
   d. provide nutrition
   e. prevent long-term complications
   f. care for skin graft
   g. support child and family
   h. prepare for discharge and home care
54. disorientation; tachypnea; temperature above 39.5° C; hypothermia; and distention of abdomen or development of intestinal ileus
55. Protection
56. F
57. sufficient exposure to cool the tissues to the point that ice crystals begin to form in interstitial spaces of superficial and deep structures, resulting in variable degrees of tissue loss and function.

Section IV A

1.
   a. potential for infection related to denuded skin, presence of pathogenic organisms
   b. altered nutrition: less than body requirements related to increased catabolism, loss of appetite
   c. impaired physical mobility related to pain, impaired joint movement
   d. body image disturbance related to perception of appearance and mobility
   e. altered family processes related to situational crisis
2.
   a. provides a soothing film that reduces external stimuli
   b. provides a palliative anti-inflammatory effect
   c. prevents autoinoculation and secondary infection
   d. helps to cool the skin by evaporation, relieve itching and inflammation, and cleanse the area by loosening and removing crusts and debris
   e. increases the penetration of the medication by promoting moisture retention, nonevap-

oration of the vehicle, and maceration of the epidermis

Section IV B

1. the identification of potential milk sensitivity and appropriate counseling
2.
   a. chronic pain related to intense pruritus
   b. impaired skin integrity related to eczematous lesions
   c. potential for infection related to risk of secondary infection of primary lesions
   d. sleep pattern disturbances related to pruritis
   e. altered family processes related to child's discomfort and lengthy therapy
3. promote healing

Section IV C

1. The nurse assessed Sean's skin and noted the presence of a rash on the convex surfaces of the diaper area.
2. the wetness, pH, and fecal irritants
3.
   a. do change diapers as soon as they become wet
   b. do expose the area to light and air
   c. do not use rubber pants
   d. do clean the area well after each soiling
   e. do use an occlusive ointment

Section IV D

1. Because of their social nature and proximity to other children
2. The crawling insect and the insect's saliva on the skin
3. Lindane (Kwell)
4.
   a. educational
   b. reinfestation-prevention
5. The pediculicide is not effective against nits. Therefore, it is necessary to retreat in order to eliminate newly hatched lice.

Section IV E

1.
   a. monitoring vital signs frequently
   b. observing for signs of overhydration
   c. being alert for altered behavior or sensorium
2. You determine the normal output for a child of your patient's age, then compare the normal output to your patient's output.
3. Infection is a leading cause of death in the

patient with thermal injury and is a serious complication. Adhering to sterile technique lessens the chance of infection.
4. Altered nutrition: less than body requirements related to loss of appetite.
5. Constipation is a frequent complication of immobility. Because the patient is probably on bed rest, it is important to monitor bowel function to prevent the bowel from getting impacted.
6. The family demonstrates an understanding of the needs of the child (diet, rest, and activity), demonstrates the wound care, and sets realistic goals.

Chapter 30

Question   Answer

Section III

1.
   a. significant loss of muscle strength, endurance, and muscle mass
   b. bone demineralization leading to osteoporosis
   c. loss of joint mobility and contractures
2. participate in his or her own care
3.
   a. damage to the soft tissue, subcutaneous structures, and muscle
   b. occurs when the force of stress on the ligament is so great that it displaces the normal position of the opposing bone ends or the bone end to its socket
   c. occurs when trauma to a joint is so severe that a ligament is partially or completely torn or stretched by the force created as a joint is twisted or wrenched, often accompanied by damage to associated blood vessels, muscles, tendons, and nerves
   d. microscopic tear to the musculotendinous unit; has features in common with sprains
4.
   a. Rest
   b. Ice
   c. Compression
   d. Elevation
5.
   a. bends—a child's flexible bone can be bent 45° or more before breaking
   b. buckle fracture—compression of the porous bone produces a buckle, or torus, fracture
   c. greenstick fracture—occurs when a bone is angulated beyond the limits of bending
   d. complete fracture—those types that divide the bone fragments

6.
  a. reduction–to regain alignment and length.
  b. immobilization–to retain alignment and length.
  c. to restore function to the injured parts.
7. traction; closed manipulation; casting
8. pain, swelling, discoloration of exposed portions, lack of pulsation and warmth, or inability to move the exposed parts
9.
  a. to fatigue the involved muscle and reduce muscle spasm so that bones can be realigned
  b. to position the distal and proximal bone ends in desired realignment to promote satisfactory bone healing
  c. to immobilize the fracture site until realignment has been achieved and sufficient healing has taken place to permit casting or splinting
10.
  a. manual traction
  b. skin traction
  c. skeletal traction
11.
  a. 5
  b. 3
  c. 4
  d. 2
  e. 1
12. A severed part should be wrapped lightly in a clean cloth or gauze saturated with normal saline and sealed in a watertight plastic bag.
13.
  a. acetabular dysplasia or preluxation
  b. subluxation
  c. dislocation
14. Ortolani; Barlow
15.
  a. 4
  b. 1
  c. 2
  d. 3
16.
  a. correction of the deformity
  b. maintenance of the correction
  c. follow-up observation to avert possible recurrence
17. heterogenous inherited disorders; connective
18.
  a. avascular
  b. fragmentation or revascularization
  c. reparative
  d. regenerative
19.
  a. structural
  b. functional

20. external or internal fixation techniques
21. Bracing
22. Traction
23. Stryker frame; bed
24. The advantage to this procedure is that the patient is able to ambulate within a few days, and no postoperative immobilization is required. The disadvantage is the possibility of spinal nerve damage.
25. infectious process of bone; exogenous; hematogenous
26. intravenous therapy; antibiotic
27. bed rest; immobilized
28. spine; hip
29. osteogenic sarcoma; Ewing sarcoma
30.
  a. arises from bone-forming mesenchyme giving rise to malignant osteoid tissue
  b. arises in the narrow spaces of the bone rather than in osseous tissue
  c. radical surgical amputation followed by intensive chemotherapy
  d. intensive radiation of the involved bone combined with chemotherapy
31. prosthesis
32. negative
33. stiffness, swelling, tenderness, painful to touch or relatively painless, warm to touch (seldom red), loss of motion, characteristic morning stiffness or "gelling" on arising in morning or after inactivity
34.
  a. Growth is retarded during active disease.
  b. Corticosteroid therapy is a contributing factor.
35.
  a. to preserve joint function
  b. to prevent physical deformities
  c. to relieve symptoms without therapeutic harm
36.
  a. Nonsteroidal antiinflammatory drugs
  b. slower-acting antirheumatic drugs
  c. cytotoxic drugs
  d. corticosteroids
37. Corticosteroids are not the drug of choice because of their chronic and serious side effects.
38. A chronic inflammatory disease of the collagen or supporting tissues.
39. an erythematous blush, or an outbreak of scaly erythematous patches, that appears over the bridge of the nose and symmetrically extends to each cheek, and that may extend to the scalp, neck, chest, and extremities. It is called a "butterfly" rash, photosensitivity.
40. the presence of renal involvement and consequent kidney failure

41.
    a. to reverse the autoimmune and inflammatory processes
    b. to prevent exacerbations and complications
42. The principal drugs are corticosteroids.
43. to help the child and family adjust to the limitations and treatments of the disease and to prevent exacerbations and complications
44. The exact relationship between SLE and rest is unclear, but fatigue or sudden exertion brings about a relapse of symptoms.

Section IV A

1.
    a. impaired physical mobility related to mechanical restrictions, physical disability
    b. high risk for impaired skin integrity related to immobility, therapeutic appliances
    c. potential for trauma related to impaired mobility
    d. diversional activity deficit related to impaired mobility, musculoskeletal impairment, confinement to hospital or home
    e. altered family processes related to a child with disability
2.
    a. prevent physical complications
    b. prevent psychologic complications
    c. provide appropriate diversional activities
    d. support child and family
3. signs of irritation, redness, or evidence of pressure on skin

Section IV B

1.
    a. Keep the extremity elevated on pillows for the first day.
    b. Avoid indenting the cast until it is thoroughly dry.
    c. Encourage frequent rest for a few days, keeping the injured extremity elevated while resting.
    d. Avoid allowing the affected limb to hang down for any length of time.
2.
    a. Do not allow child to put anything in cast.
    b. Keep clear path for ambulation.
    c. Use crutches appropriately.

Section IV C

1.
    a. Understand function of traction.

    b. Check desired line of pull frequently to maintain alignment.
    c. Check function of component parts.
    d. Make sure ropes move freely through pulleys.
    e. Make sure weights hang free.
    f. Maintain total body alignment.
    g. Do not remove traction.
2. potential for injury related to immobility due to traction
3. bleeding; inflammation; or infection

Section IV D

1.
    a. leg shortening
    b. asymmetry of the thigh and gluteal fold
    c. limited abduction
    d. positive Ortolani test
    e. positive Barlow test
2. early; age; dysplasia
3.
    a. maintain correct position of hip in acetabulum
    b. prevent complications related to wearing corrective device
    c. assist family in adapting routine nurturing activities to accommodate corrective device
4.
    a. Teach parents to apply and maintain the reduction device.
    b. Assess skin under harness for irritation daily.
    c. Avoid use of powders and lotions.
    d. Caution against unsupervised adjustment of harness.
    e. Help devise means for maintaining cleanliness.
    f. Teach positioning of child for normal activities of daily living.
    g. Provide appropriate stimulation and activities for age within limitation of harness.

Section IV E

1.
    a. body image disturbance related to the defect in body structure
    b. self-esteem disturbance related to immobility
2.
    a. accentuate positive aspects of appearance
    b. encourage Jane to wear attractive clothes and hairstyle
    c. emphasize positive long-term outcome
    d. help devise positive ways to deal with reactions of others
3. opioids administered through patient-controlled analgesia (PCA)

Section IV F

1. He would appear very ill, would be irritable, and would have an elevated temperature, rapid pulse and signs of dehydration. He would complain of localized tenderness, increased warmth, and diffuse swelling over the involved bone. The extremity would be painful, especially upon movement, and the child would hold it in semiflexion.

2.
   a. monitor intravenous equipment
   b. monitor intravenous site
   c. determine compatibility of antibiotics before administration
   d. take measures to protect the intravenous tubing from dislodgment

Section IV G

1. joints are mobile, flexible, and free of deformity
2. altered nutrition: potential for more than body requirements related to decreased mobility
3.
   a. hyperventilation—a sign of acidosis
   b. bleeding—from decreased clotting capacity
   c. tinnitus—sign of cranial nerve VIII involvement
   d. undue drowsiness—may indicate CNS depression

Chapter 31

Question	Answer

Section III

1. a nonspecific term applied to disorders characterized by impaired movement and posture and early onset. It is nonprogressive and may be accompanied by intellectual and language deficits.
2. no
3.
   a. Spastic cerebral palsy—hypertonicity with poor control of posture, balance, and coordinated motion
   b. Dyskinetic cerebral palsy—abnormal involuntary movements
   c. Ataxic cerebral palsy—wide-based gait, rapid repetitive movements performed poorly
   d. Mixed-type cerebral palsy—a combination of spasticity and athetosis
   e. Rigid, tremor, and atonic types of cerebral palsy—deformities, lack of active movement
4.
   a. delayed gross motor development

   b. abnormal motor performance
   c. alterations of muscle tone
   d. abnormal postures
   e. reflex abnormalities
   f. associated disabilities
5. may or may not be present
6.
   a. to establish locomotion, communication, and self-help
   b. to gain optimum appearance and integration of motor functions
   c. to correct associated defects as effectively as possible
   d. to provide educational opportunities adapted to the needs and capabilities of the individual child
7. physical therapy
8. d
9. b
10. muscle fibers; progressive weakness and wasting of skeletal muscles with increasing disability and deformity
11. muscle groups affected, age of onset, rate or progression, and inheritance patterns
12. pseudohypertrophic muscular dystrophy or Duchenne muscular dystrophy
13. respiratory tract infection or cardiac failure
14. Contractures and deformities
15. to maintain function in unaffected muscles for as long as possible
16. acute polyneuropathy in which motor dysfunction predominates over sensory disturbance and in which there is bilateral facial paresis or paralysis and occasionally weakness of the bulbar and respiratory musculature.
17. assisted ventilation
18. an acute, preventable, and often fatal disease caused by an exotoxin produced by the anaerobic, spore-forming, gram-positive bacillus, *Clostridium tetani.*
19. Progressive stiffness and tenderness of muscles in neck and jaw. Characteristic difficulty in opening the mouth. Facial muscle spasm causes risus sardonicus.
20. immune status; injury
21. human tetanus immune globulin (TIG)
22.
   a. provide a quiet environment that reduces external stimulation from sound, light, and touch
   b. administer the prescribed sedatives or muscle relaxants
23. ingestion of spores or vegetative cells of *C. botulinum* and the subsequent release of the toxin from organisms colonizing the gastrointestinal tract.

24. honey; light or dark corn syrup

25. history, physical examination, and laboratory detection of fecal toxin

26.

    a. complete or partial paralysis of the lower extremities

    b. no functional use of any of the four extremities

Section IV A

1.

    a. establish locomotion and communication

    b. encourage self-help

    c. facilitate acquisition of educational opportunities adapted to needs and capabilities of the child

    d. promote a positive self-image in the child

    e. support the family in its efforts to meet the needs of the child

    f. care for the child during hospitalization

2.

    a. impaired physical mobility related to neuromuscular impairment

    b. bathing/hygiene, dressing, grooming, feeding, toileting self-care deficits related to physical disability

    c. potential for injury related to physical disability, neuromuscular impairment, perceptual and cognitive impairment

    d. impaired verbal communication

    e. fatigue related to increased energy expenditure

    f. body image disturbance related to perception of disability

    g. altered family processes related to a child with a lifelong disability

Section IV B

1.

    a. prevent damage to the myelomeningocele sac

    b. prevent complications

    c. support and educate family

2.

    a. The myelomeningocele sac sustains no damage.

    b. The child exhibits no evidence of complications.

    c. The family members discuss their feelings and concerns and participate in the infant's care.

Section IV C

1. help parents develop a balance between limiting the child's activity because of muscular weakness and allowing him to accomplish things by himself

2. encouraging parents to seek genetic counseling

Section IV D

1. to prevent complications of the disease

2.

    a. observe for difficulty in swallowing and for respiratory involvement

    b. take frequent vital signs

    c. monitor level of consciousness

    d. maintain good postural alignment

    e. change position frequently

    f. perform passive range of motion every 4 hours

    g. ensure adequate nutrition

    h. provide bowel and bladder care to prevent constipation and urine retention

Section IV E

1.

    a. prevention of complications

    b. maintenance of function

2. interdisciplinary